Hopkin, Karen.

Understanding cystic
  fibrosis.

$12.00

DATE			

Understanding Health and Sickness Series
Miriam Bloom, Ph.D.
General Editor

Understanding Cystic Fibrosis

Karen Hopkin, Ph.D.

University Press of Mississippi
Jackson

Library of Congress Cataloging-in-Publication Data

Hopkin, Karen.
     Understanding cystic fibrosis / Karen Hopkin.
          p.   cm.—(Understanding health and sickness series)
     Includes index.
     ISBN 0-87805-966-0 (cloth : alk. paper).—ISBN 0-87805-967-9
(pbk. : alk. paper)
     1. Cystic fibrosis—Popular works.   I. Title.   II. Series.
RC858.C95H67   1998
616.3'7—dc21   97-38646
                                                            CIP

British Library Cataloging-in-Publication data available

Contents

Acknowledgments

I would like to thank my editors at the *Journal of NIH Research*—Bruce Agnew, Carol Ezzell, and Keith Haglund—for asking me to write an article about the latest experimental treatments for cystic fibrosis (CF). That article effectively launched this book. Special thanks go to Bruce for his unwavering support and editorial guidance and to Keith for slogging through my early drafts and working tirelessly to help make the manuscript readable and for allowing me to take two days off from work to write the book.

I would also like to thank the researchers who gave of their time to help me formulate the original *JNIHR* article, which formed the backbone of chapter 7: Richard Boucher, David Bedwell, Mike Welsh, Jeff Smith, Ron Crystal, Lap-Chee Tsui, James Wilson, Paul Fischer, and Alan Smith. Special thanks go to Michael Rock of the University of Wisconsin Children's Hospital in Madison for taking time out of his busy schedule—and his vacation—to review the manuscript carefully and to Lap-Chee Tsui, who somehow managed to read through the book and offer insightful comments while traveling between conferences. I am also grateful to Scott Tebbutt of the University of Otago in Dunedin, New Zealand, for his helpful discussions on CF animal studies and for pointing me toward the most informative CF Web sites.

Special thanks also go to the good folks at University Press of Mississippi: to Miriam Bloom for her confidence and her thoughtful suggestions on an early draft of my first chapter and to Seetha Srinivasan for her encouragement and her patience in waiting for the final manuscript. I thank Regan Tuder for her clear illustrations and Jeff Smith of the University of Iowa College of Medicine in Iowa City for permission to reproduce the striking electron micrographs of lung cells.

Thanks go as well to the people at the CF Foundation who directed me to the most exciting research and supplied me with a great deal of background information on the disease—diagnosis, treatments, and expectations for the future.

Finally, very special thanks to Camille Collett, friend and colleague, for her support, encouragement, and constant cajoling.

Introduction

Cystic fibrosis (CF) used to be considered a childhood disease, because people born with it rarely lived to reach adolescence. Now, with marked improvement in treatments—from physiotherapy and antibiotics that keep the lungs clear of mucus and microbes to enzyme supplements that aid digestion—many people with CF live into their thirties and beyond. The discovery of the gene responsible for CF has given scientists a better understanding of how the disease impairs the function of the lungs, pancreas, sweat glands, and other organs. And researchers and clinicians are now turning this enhanced knowledge into specific new treatments that may someday lead to a cure for CF.

In the United States, about 900 children with CF are born each year. The disease occurs in about 1 of every 3,300 white newborns and 1 of every 17,000 African-American newborns. Cystic fibrosis is the most common genetic disorder in the white population, and the discovery of the CF gene has opened the way for doctors to develop genetic tests that will allow accurate, early diagnosis.

This book, written for people with CF and for their friends, families, and health care workers, contains the latest information on the diagnosis, treatment, and biology of the disease. Scientists around the world had engaged in a heated race to find the CF gene, and its discovery was one of the most valued prizes in medicine. Because the disease is caused by mutations in a single gene, researchers are trying to develop methods of inserting healthy copies of the gene into the lungs of people with CF. Since researchers identified the CF gene in 1989, about 140 people with CF in the United States have received experimental gene therapy. None of these studies has gone on long enough to indicate whether gene therapy strategies will ultimately prove successful at relieving the most serious problems associated with CF.

The book begins with a brief description of CF and a discussion of how the disease is inherited. We review some basic genetics and show how to calculate the odds that a couple will have a child with CF. The first chapter also describes how mutations in the gene that causes CF impair the function of specialized cells in the lungs, pancreas, and other organs. We then consider where CF may have originated and why the disease might still be around.

In chapter 2, we look at the history of CF—how doctors first recognized it as a disease and how their studies and observations led to current diagnoses and treatments. The next two chapters tell about the race for the discovery of the CF gene and about how defects in that gene affect the body's organs. In chapter 5, we examine the most common treatments for CF, including chest physiotherapy, antibiotics, enzyme supplements, exercise, and lung transplant operations. The following chapter describes how people with CF and their friends and families cope psychologically with this fatal disease, and also discusses how genetic counselors can help carriers and parents understand the risk of having a child with CF so they can make decisions about family planning. In the final chapter, we review the current state of CF research and relate the types of treatments that scientists hope may someday lead to a cure.

Finally, the appendix lists organizations and other sources that can provide information and support, including sites on the Internet offering forums where people with CF can engage in discussions and locate information. Addresses are given for newsletters and CF centers around the country; these will also help anyone interested in CF find the answers to their questions.

Many fine books on CF are available. In preparing this book, I consulted *Cystic Fibrosis: The Facts* by Ann Harris and Maurice Saper (Oxford University Press, 1995) and *A Parent's Guide to Cystic Fibrosis* by Burton Shapiro and Ralph Heussner (University of Minnesota Press, 1991). Other titles are listed on the CF Web home page at *http://www.ai.mit.edu/people/mernst/cf.*

Understanding Cystic Fibrosis

1. Who Gets Cystic Fibrosis and How?

Cystic fibrosis is the most common genetic disorder in the white population.

Almost every article or book about cystic fibrosis (CF) begins with a statement similar to the one above. But what exactly is a genetic disorder, and what does it mean to have such a condition? How is it passed along? And why is this one most common in whites?

People who have genetic disorders are born with them. The inherited genetic defect causes a chemical error in all the cells in their bodies. In children and adults with CF, a mistake in a single gene disables a type of protein that functions as an *ion channel*. This molecule regulates the balance of salts in a special type of cell that lines many of the body's glands. All people with genetic disorders have inherited the defective genes from their parents, who in turn had inherited them from their parents, and so on, stretching back many generations. Although people with CF have the disease from the moment of conception, the symptoms can appear at different ages and vary in severity from person to person. People with CF have difficulty breathing, and most also experience digestive problems. These and other symptoms of CF are related to the salt imbalance caused by the basic genetic defect. In any case, CF is present even before a baby is born.

An inherited disease is not contagious; it cannot be caught as if it were a cold or the flu. And because CF is caused by a genetic defect, people who have the disease cannot outgrow it but must live with it throughout their lives. The treatments currently available aim to alleviate the symptoms so that people with CF can enjoy full, active, and productive lives. As doctors learn more about the disease and how to treat it, the average life expectancy for people with CF continues to climb. In the 1950s, the median survival age for people with CF was eight years; today it is thirty.

A person with CF has inherited two copies of a defective (or *mutant*) gene—one from each parent. Someone who has only one copy of the mutant gene is called a *carrier*. Carriers are healthy individuals who never develop CF symptoms, but who can pass the disease on to their children. The gene that is defective in those with CF normally directs certain cells in the body to make a salt-regulating protein called the *cystic fibrosis transmembrane conductance regulator (CFTR)*. Because CF carriers have one normal copy of the CFTR gene, they generate enough normal CFTR protein to keep their cells healthy and functioning correctly.

The normal CFTR protein forms a molecular tunnel or channel that allows salt—specifically the chloride portion of *sodium chloride* (table salt)—to enter and exit the cell. Thousands of CFTR protein channels sit nestled in the membranes of cells that line the lungs, intestines, pancreas, sweat glands, and reproductive tract. A normal CFTR protein snakes in and out of the cell membrane, forming a pore that allows passage of chloride ions into or out of the cell. The pore of the channel normally remains closed. But when the cell needs to get rid of some salt, the shape of the CFTR protein changes and allows the pore to open briefly and let the salt pass through. When CFTR channels are defective or missing entirely—as they are in people with CF who have inherited defective CFTR genes from both parents—chloride ions and the water in which they are dissolved cannot flow properly through the cell membrane. Many cells in the body rely on such channels of one type or another to perform their biological duties. But the specialized *epithelial cells* that line the body's *exocrine glands*—those that secrete their products through ducts—rely on the CFTR channel to maintain the proper salt balance and to adjust the thickness of their secretions. Epithelial cells form thin sheets that regulate which molecules can enter a tissue or organ and which can leave.

Exocrine glands produce a variety of secretions, including sweat, tears, mucus, and the enzymes that help digest the food we eat. In people with CF, the decreased flow of salt from epithelial cells causes the exocrine glands to produce thick, sticky secretions that can plug up the ducts connecting them to the airways, the intestines, or the outside world. In the lungs, normal mucus helps to remove dust and germs from the airways. The thickened mucus produced by people with CF can make the lungs more susceptible to infection by bacteria and other microbes. In the pancreas, plugs of thickened mucus can interfere with digestion by blocking the secretion of the enzymes that help digest food. And, in the sweat glands, cells that contain mutant CFTR do not reabsorb chloride, which causes the sweat of people with CF to be especially salty. In fact, doctors measure the amount of salt in sweat as a diagnostic test for CF.

According to the Cystic Fibrosis Foundation (CFF), currently some 30,000 people in the United States have CF. Although CF is rarer in Asian Americans and Native Americans than in whites and African Americans, the disease affects virtually every race. In the United States, almost 1 person in 30 carries the gene for CF, which means that about 10 million Americans have 1 copy of the defective CF gene.

CF AND HEREDITY

"Ooooh, he has his mother's eyes!" coo the doting aunties huddled around the new infant's bassinet. "But where'd he get that mop of hair?"

Genes influence all of our physical characteristics—from hair and eye color to the shape of our ears and the length of our legs.

Some traits, such as the ability to curl one's tongue, are dictated by a single gene. Other traits are more complex and result from a combination of different genes. For example, scientists believe that 3 to 6 pairs of genes may contribute to skin color in humans. Characteristics like hair color, nose shape, and a sense of humor are also probably not the product of a single gene.

Many of the genes that contribute to complex traits— intelligence, athletic ability, or a natural talent for playing the tuba—merely confer potential. Although genes might contribute to a person's coordination and muscle development, he or she acquires the ability to sink a basketball from three-point range only after a great deal of practice; no combination of genes can code for the perfect jump shot. Even traits as seemingly straightforward as height respond to environmental influences. Individuals who possess "tall" genes might not reach full height if they do not receive proper nourishment when their bones are growing.

Regardless of how many genes influence a given trait, all genes come from an individual's parents. Genes provide cells with a detailed set of instructions encoded in the chemical sequence of a molecule called *deoxyribonucleic acid* (*DNA*). DNA acts like a long, winding piece of molecular ticker tape that contains all the information a cell needs to make the proteins necessary for it to develop into a heart cell, a bone cell, or a cell in the retina of the eye, and to carry out its specialized functions.

In a human being, scientists estimate that some 60,000 to 100,000 genes tell cells how to operate and grow. These genes, made of DNA, are stored on the chromosomes inside the nucleus of the cell. Humans have 23 pairs of chromosomes—one set of 23 from each parent. Because human chromosomes are paired, the genes along those chromosomes also come in pairs. For every gene, an individual gets one copy, called an *allele*, from the mother and one copy from the father. Genes that fall on the sex chromosomes—X and Y—are the only exceptions. Because females have two X chromosomes and males have one X and one Y, boys inherit genes on the Y chromosome only from their fathers.

What controls which genes a person will inherit? At conception, 1 sperm cell joins 1 egg. Each of these *gametes*, as they're generically called, contains 1 set of 23 chromosomes. When a sperm and an egg combine to form the embryo, they reconstitute the full complement of 46 chromosomes. All 46 chromosomes are present in every cell in the body—except for the gametes, which reduce the number back down to 23, and red blood cells, which lose their chromosomes when they mature. With half the genes coming from the egg and half from the sperm, which genes an individual inherits depends on which genes each gamete received when it formed in the testes or ovary of the parent.

Because each gamete receives only a single copy of each gene, every allele—whether it influences hair color, eye color, height, or earlobe shape—has a 50–50 chance of making it into a sperm or an egg. So genetic inheritance is based on a molecular coin toss. The same holds true for every one of the 60,000-plus genes in human beings, including the CFTR gene (fig. 1.1). In carriers who have one normal copy of the CFTR gene and one mutant copy, each gamete runs a 50 percent chance of receiving the normal gene and a 50 percent chance of receiving the defective gene.

Not all genes are equal. Some are *dominant*: inheriting a single copy of the gene will give the individual that trait. Other genes, including the mutant CFTR gene, are *recessive*: a person must inherit two mutant CFTR genes in order to have CF. Carriers who possess one normal CFTR gene are healthy and do not have CF.

Understanding that genes segregate by chance, people who know whether they carry a defective CFTR gene can easily calculate the odds that their children will be born with CF. If both parents have two normal copies of the CFTR gene, none of their children can get CF disease. If one parent is a carrier and the other parent has two normal copies of the CFTR gene, again, the children cannot inherit CF disease. (Remember, people with CF inherit two defective copies of the CFTR gene—one from each parent.) If two people with CF were able to conceive children together (which might not be easy, because males with CF are usually infertile), their children would all be born with CF because they would inherit only defective CFTR genes.

But what happens when both parents are carriers (fig. 1.2)? In genetic lingo, such individuals are referred to as *heterozygotes* because they possess a nonidentical pair of genes—one normal and one that contains a mutation. *Homozygous* individuals possess identical alleles—either two normal genes or two mutant genes.

The easiest way to figure out what to expect for the children is to begin by thinking about what kind of CFTR genes can wind up in the gametes of each of the parents. Odds are that half of the father's sperm and half of the mother's eggs will harbor the mutant CFTR gene and half will have the normal CFTR gene.

Now, consider the possible combinations. First, a sperm with a normal CFTR gene can combine with an egg with a normal CFTR gene; this child will not have CF and will not be a carrier. Second, a sperm with a mutant CFTR gene can combine with an egg with a normal CFTR gene; this child will be a carrier. Likewise, a sperm with a normal CFTR gene could couple with an egg with a mutant CFTR gene to produce a carrier. Finally, a sperm with a mutant CFTR gene can combine with an egg with a mutant CFTR gene, resulting in a fetus with CF.

Those are the only combinations possible when both parents are carriers. Given those 4 situations, the odds that a child will not have CF and will not be a carrier (homozygous normal) are 1 in 4, or 25 percent. The chances that the child will be a heterozygous carrier are 2 in 4, or 50 percent. Finally, the chances that a child will have CF is 1 in 4, again 25 percent.

Because there is no way to predict which sperm will meet with which egg at the time of conception, these odds apply to every pregnancy individually. It is not necessarily true that if a couple has four children, one will have CF or that if a couple conceives one child with CF the next three will be free of the disease.

Most healthy individuals do not know whether they carry a mutant CF gene. Few people seek the tests that would indicate

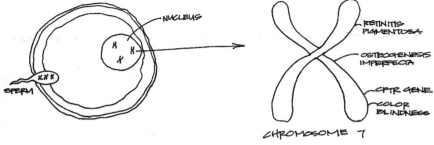

FIG. 1.1. Fertilization. When a sperm and an egg fuse, they each contribute an equal number of chromosomes to the young embryo. Although only 3 chromosomes are shown here, in humans each gamete actually contributes 23. Each chromosome carries many, many genes. Chromosome 7, which carries the gene responsible for CF, also carries genes that can contribute to color blindness, retinitis pigmentosa (a disease that causes degeneration of the retina), and osteogenesis imperfecta (a family of diseases causing fragile bones).

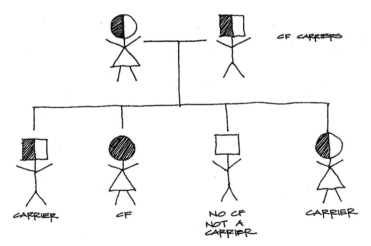

FIG. 1.2. A CF family tree. Pedigree charts can track cystic fibrosis, and the genes that cause it, through the generations. This chart represents the offspring of two parents who are CF carriers. The completely filled symbol represents a child with CF; the half-filled symbols represent carriers.

whether such a gene is present unless they know that CF runs in their family or they have already had a child with CF. If about 1 in 30 whites is a carrier, the risks of someone in the general population having a child with CF can be estimated from the following table:

One Parent	Other Parent	Odds
Known carrier	Known carrier	1 in 4
Known carrier	General population	1 in 120
Person with CF	General population	1 in 60
Sibling of CF	General population	1 in 180
General population	General population	1 in 3,600

People who have parents, siblings, or other relatives with CF can determine their risks more accurately by going to a genetic counselor and getting screened for the most common CFTR mutations. As it turns out, a defective CFTR gene may harbor any one of hundreds of different mutations that are all known to cause CF. Individuals who know whether they carry a mutant CFTR gene can make more informed decisions about planning a family or can decide whether to test their children for CF prenatally. (See chapter 6 for a more detailed discussion of genetic screening.)

WHAT EXACTLY IS A GENE?

In the late 1800s, an educated and curious Austrian monk named Gregor Mendel took it upon himself to unravel the laws of inheritance—that is, how traits are passed on from parents to their offspring. He selected peas as his experimental subject; the plants could be grown easily by the dozens in a small plot of land in the monastery garden, and more important, he could control which plants mated with which by manually removing pollen (plant sperm) from one pea plant and brushing it onto the ova-bearing pistil of another.

Mendel wondered what made some of the plants tall and others short, and why some peas were yellow and some green, some wrinkled and some smooth. By mating scores of pea plants, Mendel could follow their patterns of inheritance from one generation to the next. He determined that individual traits were inherited separately—a plant could be tall with green peas or tall with yellow peas, or it could be short with wrinkled peas or short with smooth peas.

He also found that some traits are dominant and some recessive: when he mated a plant with smooth peas with a plant with wrinkled peas, the first generation of offspring all had smooth peas. Like the gene for CF, the wrinkled gene is recessive. And though the first generation of plants had smooth peas, they each carried one copy of the gene for wrinkled peas, which they had inherited from the wrinkled-pea parent. When these first-generation offspring are mated with one another, one-quarter of their progeny have wrinkled peas—just as the CF carriers have a 25 percent chance of having children with CF. By doing the math, Mendel realized that for every trait, each parent contributed one hereditary "factor"—a unit we now call a gene. Although some science historians believe that Mendel may have fudged some of his numbers (they were too good—in real experiments the ratios never come out *exactly* right), his ideas formed the basis of modern genetics.

What are genes made of? Cells contain 4 different types of large molecules—proteins, nucleic acids (including DNA), fats, and carbohydrates. Early on, scientists believed that proteins carried genetic information from generation to generation. Proteins were appealing candidates for genetic material because they are composed of long strings of 20 different amino acids. DNA, on the other hand, consists of repeating sequences of only 4 chemicals called *nucleotide bases—adenine*, *guanine*, *cytosine*, and *thymine*—A, G, C, and T for short. Scientists initially thought that DNA was too simple a molecule to carry the blueprint for life. If the nucleotides and amino acids are like the letters of the alphabet, scientists reasoned, proteins could spell a larger variety of words than DNA. And certainly genes, which influence everything from hair color to mathematical ability, convey a rich variety of information.

It wasn't until the 1940s that Oswald Avery, Colin MacLeod, and Maclyn McCarty of Rockefeller University in New York City offered the first proof that DNA carries and transmits genetic information. The researchers were working with a type of bacteria called *pneumococcus*. When these microbes are grown on a culture dish, they form little colonies. Some colonies appear smooth and shiny; others look rough and wrinkled. The Rockefeller researchers found that if they took DNA purified from a smooth colony and introduced it into a culture of pneumococcus that formed rough colonies, they could convince the rough bacteria to form smooth colonies. Just like the smooth peas, pneumococcus exposed to the smooth genes formed smooth colonies, and it was DNA—not protein—that carried the instructions.

An understanding of how DNA carried and passed along genetic information fell into place a decade later. In the 1950s, James Watson and Francis Crick deduced DNA's double-helical structure. The genetic material consists of two strands of DNA that wind around one another forming a sort of molecular spiral staircase. The rungs are made of complementary pairs of nucleotide bases, the twisting backbone of groups of sugar and phosphate (fig. 1.3).

The sequence of the nucleotide bases—A, T, C, and G—forms a genetic code that dictates and controls the production of all the proteins in the cell. Specialized enzymes in the cell decipher the code and synthesize the proper proteins. The "words" of the code are each made of three nucleotide-base "letters." These nucleotide triplets tell the cell machinery which amino acid to insert into the growing protein. For example, the string ATG CGT AGT GGT CTT TGG TAG encodes a protein fragment with the amino acid sequence: arginine-serine-glycine-leucine-tryptophan. The first ATG serves as a flag that indicates the start of a protein sequence. The final TAG, called a stop

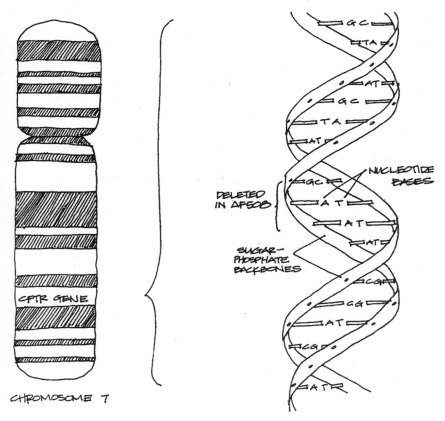

FIG. I.3. What's a gene? The CFTR gene lies on the long arm of human chromosome 7. Like all genes, CFTR is made of two intertwined strands of DNA. The order of the nucleotide bases—the rungs of this spiraling molecular staircase—dictate the amino-acid sequence of the protein that the cell will make from the CFTR gene. The most common mutation in people with CF, called ΔF508, directs the cell to make a CFTR channel protein missing one amino acid—phenylalanine 508.

codon, signals the cell machinery that the sequence is finished. Almost all of the amino acids can be encoded by more than one triplet. For example, TCT, TCC, TCA, and TCG all code for serine.

DNA has two jobs. It passes information from parent to offspring. But it also dictates the activity in our cells and tells cells what proteins to make. How DNA makes proteins is one of the most extensively studied processes in biology. Molecular machinery in the cell nucleus transcribes the DNA code into a related messenger molecule, *ribonucleic acid* (*RNA*). The messenger RNA leaves the nucleus and goes into the cytoplasm of the cell, where other specialized molecules translate its information into proteins, including CFTR. The whole process is so important and so clearly established that scientists refer to it as the central dogma: DNA → RNA → Protein. So, what do proteins like CFTR do?

WHAT IS CFTR?

Proteins form the main architecture of the cell and also do most of the cellular work. They hasten chemical reactions and carry chemical messages from one cell to the next. Once they're made, proteins migrate to different locations in the cell, depending on their duties. Proteins that signal other cells are exported to the extracellular horizons that lie beyond the membrane encasing each cell. Some proteins spread throughout the cytoplasm inside the cell, laying the foundation for the cell's structural meshwork, the *cytoskeleton*. Others remain in the nucleus where they help to regulate DNA synthesis. Still others find their way to the cell membrane where they perform their molecular duties.

CFTR is a protein that gets shipped to the membrane, where it acts as a channel through which chloride ions enter and exit the cell. CFTR is most active in the cells that line exocrine glands, particularly the pancreatic ducts, sweat glands, mucous glands in the lungs, and the ducts of the male reproductive tract. When CFTR is absent or defective, these glands lose their ability to regulate the flow of salt into and out of their cells. In the lungs, abnormal concentrations of salt cause the mucous layer that coats the airways to become sticky and thick. In the sweat glands, normal CFTR controls the reabsorption of salt into the body. Losing too much salt in sweat can throw off the normal functioning of cells throughout the body. That's why runners and other athletes guzzle sports drinks that contain electrolytes, which are essentially salts to replace what the body has lost in the form of sweat during heavy exercise.

In 1989, scientists led by Lap-Chee Tsui and John Riordan of the Toronto Hospital for Sick Children and Francis Collins of the Howard Hughes Medical Institute at the University of Michigan in Ann Arbor identified the gene that causes CF. Before that, scientists had not been sure that the CFTR protein was a chloride channel. After the researchers determined the sequence of the CFTR gene—identifying the proper order of the As, Ts, Gs, and Cs it contains—they figured out the amino-acid sequence of the CFTR protein. They then ran the amino-acid sequence through a computer program that predicts the potential structure of the protein. Because scientists knew that CF disease was associated with defective chloride channel activity, they suspected that the CFTR protein might be a channel. But CFTR's function was not confirmed until the normal CFTR gene was put into test cells; scientists then determined that those cells produce normal CFTR protein and exhibit chloride channel activity. (See chapter 3 for further discussion of how scientists discovered the CFTR gene, what they think the CFTR protein looks like, and how it functions.)

WHAT MUTATIONS CAUSE CF?

According to Dr. Tsui, more than 700 different mutations in the CFTR gene can cause CF. Some mutations direct the cell to manufacture a dysfunctional CFTR protein; others cause it to be missing entirely. About 90 percent of people with CF carry the most common mutation, called *delta F508*, or ΔF508 (fig. 1.3). This mutation directs the cell to produce a CFTR protein that is missing a single amino acid—a *phenylalanine* (F) at position 508 in a protein made of 1480 amino acids. How can such a small change cause such a serious disease? The loss of the phenylalanine residue somehow prevents the CFTR protein from being folded into the proper shape and inserted into the cell membrane.

Other mutations in the CFTR gene produce fragments of CFTR proteins that are too small to function properly or CFTR proteins that do not respond appropriately to chemical cues inside the cell. Does the type of CFTR mutation a person is born with influence the severity of the disease? This question is not easy to answer. To determine whether particular mutations correlate with milder or more severe CF symptoms, scientists need to compare the disease course of many individuals with the same genetic mistakes in the CFTR gene. Collecting enough data on the mutations that are not as common as ΔF508 has proven difficult. In the families that have been studied extensively, the complexity of CF makes for some conflicting results. Siblings, even identical twins, who possess the same CFTR mutations may not experience the same degree of severity of symptoms because of nongenetic factors, such as the environment.

Generally speaking, people with the ΔF508 mutation usually have a more severe form of CF. In addition to chronic problems with the lungs, these people almost always experience digestive difficulties related to the pancreas. When the pancreatic ducts become plugged with mucus, the digestive enzymes produced by the pancreas cannot make it to the intestine where they are needed to digest food. But whether patients with CF will have milder or more severe respiratory problems is hard to predict from their CFTR mutation. Some evidence suggests that when CFTR mutations affect the conductance of the channels, by causing the cells to produce a mutant CFTR protein that permits fewer chloride ions to pass through than a normal CFTR channel would, the result is sometimes a milder form of CF.

Scientists studying a mouse model of CF find that, in addition to mutations in the CFTR gene, the activity of other genes may influence the course of CF disease. Normal mice have a gene that's very similar to the human CFTR gene. To learn more about what happens in cells that do not have any CFTR channels, researchers have generated mice that do not produce CFTR proteins. Like humans with CF, some of the mice are less sick than others. And the scientists found that in the mice with milder symptoms another chloride channel protein may be activated which helps to compensate for the loss of CFTR. If scientists could figure out how to coax other chloride channels to be more active in the cells lacking CFTR, they might be able to develop a drug treatment that would effectively alleviate the symptoms of CF.

WHERE DO MUTATIONS COME FROM?

Genetic mistakes can crop up at various times during evolution. Mutant genes get copied, distributed to the gametes, and passed along, from parent to offspring, through the generations. Some scientists believe that CF may have arisen in the Middle East more than 50,000 years ago and may have spread across Europe as farmers began to migrate to the northwest at the end of the Stone Age, some 10,000 years ago.

Although the origins of the mutations that cause CF are still open to debate, in general, mutations can arise spontaneously or following exposure to radiation or chemicals that damage the nucleotide bases of DNA. No machine is perfect, including the cellular machinery that makes the copies of an individual's DNA which will get distributed to the gametes and be passed on via sexual reproduction. If the DNA-replicating machinery falters or slips even the tiniest bit when it's copying a gene sequence, it might produce a DNA copy that is missing a nucleotide base. And sometimes the machinery just makes a simple mistake and inserts the wrong nucleotide base into a gene sequence. The cellular enzymes that replicate DNA make, on average, 1 mistake for every 10,000,000 to 1,000,000,000 bases they copy. Generating 1 error every billion or so bases might seem insignificant, but, in humans, this spontaneous mutation rate could cause 1 or 2 mutations to crop up in every 100,000 gametes—sperm or egg—made by an individual. If males release about 350 million sperm cells in every ejaculate, they could introduce new mutations to their offspring during any mating. Of course, not all mutations are bad or at least not as bad as the mistakes that cause CF. Others may be so bad that they kill an embryo before it has a chance to develop.

X-rays and ultraviolet radiation can also damage DNA bases, as do chemicals such as the preservative formaldehyde. The damage can make a nucleotide base in the DNA sequence look like a different base, fooling the replication machinery into making a copying error. And, in some cases, if the base is damaged enough to be unrecognizable, the cellular machinery will take a guess and randomly incorporate any base at hand into the sequence. Many times, when such mistakes are made, the cell detects and repairs them. But sometimes the repair systems themselves can introduce errors into the DNA sequence.

The human CFTR gene is huge, consisting of about 250,000 nucleotide bases. If a single mistake in each of the 2 copies of a person's CFTR gene—altering a total of 2 nucleotide bases in 500,000—can cause such a devastating disease, perhaps it's surprising, mathematically speaking, that more people don't have CF.

Why did the mutant CFTR gene remain in the population? If people who inherit two copies of the mutant gene get terribly sick, why didn't the mutation just disappear? Some scientists believe that a single copy of the defective CFTR gene might have provided some type of survival advantage to its carriers—a situation that kept the gene alive in the populations that inherited it.

HOW COULD A DEFECTIVE CFTR GENE BE BENEFICIAL?

Two mutated copies of the CFTR gene cause CF, a serious illness that often claims the lives of affected individuals at a young age. So what possible benefit could there be in possessing a single copy of a defective CFTR gene? Scientists think that a mutant CF gene might protect carriers from cholera.

The idea that a recessive disease-causing allele can protect its carriers from some other, seemingly unrelated disease is not a new one. For decades scientists have known that two mutant sickle cell genes cause sickle cell disease, but that one mutant gene can protect a carrier from contracting malaria. (For more information about sickle cell disease, see *Understanding Sickle Cell Disease* by Miriam Bloom, University Press of Mississippi, 1995.)

How might a mutant CFTR gene protect a carrier against cholera? Many pathogenic bacteria, including *Vibrio cholerae*, kill people by releasing a toxin that disrupts cellular chloride channels, causing severe diarrhea, electrolyte imbalances, and a rapid loss of body fluid. So people who have fewer chloride channels—people with a mutant CFTR gene—should be less susceptible to the deadly effects of cholera toxin. To confirm this idea, scientists again turned to the mouse. Mutant mice that have one normal copy of the mouse CFTR gene and one mutant copy produce half the amount of functional CFTR channel proteins in the cells that line their intestines. When these mice are exposed to cholera toxin, they lose half as much fluid and salt as their counterparts with two normal copies of the CFTR gene. These results support the theory that mutant CF genes have remained in the gene pool because they protect carriers from cholera.

2. CF: History, Symptoms, and Diagnosis

Woe to that child which when kissed on the forehead tastes salty.
He is bewitched and soon must die.

Anonymous

This gloomy bit of northern European folklore from the eighteenth or nineteenth century almost certainly refers to children with CF, who taste salty when kissed because they lose a higher than normal amount of salt in their sweat. Doctors take advantage of this hallmark symptom of CF to diagnose the disease, particularly in infants and children; the sweat test remains the quickest and most accurate means of making such a diagnosis. Obviously, however, children with CF are not bewitched. And now, thanks to improvements in the treatment of the disease, people with CF are not fated to die before they reach adulthood, but live, on average, past the age of thirty, with increasing numbers surviving into their sixties. (In 1971, only 11 percent of the patients registered at CF treatment centers in the United States were over eighteen. By 1994, that figure had tripled, and it continues to rise.)

CF has been in the human population for centuries, but doctors did not recognize it as a unique disease until the 1930s. Why the delay? And how did physicians finally figure out how to diagnose and treat children with CF?

CF: A BRIEF HISTORY

The earliest advances in understanding and treating CF were made not in the laboratory, where so much research takes place today, but in the clinic. Physicians who spent countless hours at the bedsides of infants and children with CF provided the first big insights into the nature of the disease.

By the early 1900s, a number of articles in the medical literature had detailed cases of newborn infants with pancreatic disorders that impaired their ability to properly digest food. These reports probably provided the first clinical descriptions of CF.

But doctors did not yet recognize CF as a distinct disease, instead viewing the various symptoms—difficulty digesting food, chronic lung infections—as belonging to separate, unrelated disorders. In papers published in 1928 and in 1936, the Swiss pediatrician Guido Fanconi described children with pancreatic problems that were probably caused by CF. But physicians still were not sure whether digestive disorders and recurring bronchitis could be part of the same disease.

It was the widespread use of antibiotics in the 1940s and 1950s which helped doctors to see that the respiratory and digestive symptoms were indeed connected. Children who came to the clinic with pneumonia and with digestive problems caused by bacterial infections responded well to treatment with antibiotics, fighting off the infections and regaining their health. But doctors found that some children who had recurrent chest infections and digestive problems could not be cured by antibiotics. The drugs sometimes provided temporary relief, but the children eventually fell ill again. The infections reappeared because the antibiotics did not treat the underlying problem: the disease that would soon be called cystic fibrosis.

In 1938, Dorothy Andersen of Columbia University published the first comprehensive description of CF as a specific disorder. She reviewed the case histories of 49 infants and children with a unique combination of digestive and respiratory symptoms and presented a careful study of how the disease affected their organs. When Andersen performed autopsies on the children, she noted that their pancreases appeared scarred and that often their lungs were infected and damaged. Andersen named the disease *cystic fibrosis of the pancreas*, because the pancreas in affected individuals is riddled with patches of fibrous scar tissue that surround fluid-filled spaces called cysts.

Andersen continued to study CF and, in 1946, she recommended treating affected children with a high-calorie, high-protein, low-fat diet, supplemented with digestive enzymes purified from the pancreases of animals. Prescribing enzyme supplements to help people with CF digest their food remains a staple in the CF treatment protocols to this day. Because enzyme supplements are so effective, the digestive problems associated with CF are the most easily treated symptoms.

Two years later, Andersen and her colleagues discovered that CF patients were prone to have recurring chest infections caused by a particular type of bacteria called *Staphylococcus*. *Staphyloccocus* bacteria, particularly a species called *S. aureus*, are aggressive microbes that also infect healthy individuals. Before effective antibiotics were discovered, repeated chest infections with *S. aureus* often killed children with CF before they reached the age of seven.

By the late 1940s, physicians had realized that a defect in mucus secretion throughout the body could explain many of the symptoms of CF. They noted that the ducts in several organs of children with CF become clogged with unusually thick mucus. In the pancreas, the ducts that allow digestive enzymes to pass into the small intestine become blocked with mucus; in the lungs, the bronchial tubes become obstructed, impairing breathing and encouraging infection. But it was years before scientists determined that a defective channel protein that controls the flow of chloride ions was responsible for the thick mucus in these different organ systems.

While doctors were studying the physiology of CF, geneticists were tracking its inheritance pattern. Throughout the late 1940s and early 1950s, scientists studying families with CF determined that the disease is caused by mistakes in a single recessive gene. They found that children with CF must have inherited two defective copies of the gene responsible for CF (now known as the CFTR gene)—one from each parent. As we learned in chapter 1, children with one normal copy of the CFTR gene do not have CF.

A heat wave that blanketed New York City in the summer of 1952 provided doctors with the clue they needed to develop an effective test for diagnosing CF. As the city streets baked, hospitals admitted an unusual number of children with CF; they had become dehydrated more quickly than their unaffected playmates. That's when Paul di Sant-Agnese and his colleagues at Columbia University College of Physicians and Surgeons realized that children with CF have particularly salty sweat—an observation that allowed them to develop a diagnostic test. Once physiologists Lewis Gibson and Robert Cooke of the Johns Hopkins University Medical School in Baltimore had developed an effective method for collecting sweat, doctors began using the sweat test to diagnose children with CF.

WHEN DID CFTR ENTER THE PICTURE?

Progress in understanding the molecular basis of CF lagged behind the advances made in the clinic, and insights into the cellular defects responsible for the disease's symptoms didn't occur until the 1980s. By that time, scientists realized that the epithelial cells lining the organs impaired by CF do not function properly. Thin sheets of epithelial cells within organs such as the lungs and pancreas regulate which molecules can enter and which can leave. Epithelial cells often secrete mucus that keeps the internal surfaces of the organs lubricated and allows nutrients and gases to dissolve and pass through.

Two different sets of experiments led scientists to discover that the epithelial cells in patients with CF did not permit salt to properly pass into or out of certain organs. Paul Quinton of the University of California at Riverside found that in people with CF, epithelial cells lining the ducts of the sweat glands failed to take up chloride from the gland. Sweat is produced by cells at the base of the sweat gland and then flows to the surface of the skin through a thin duct. Epithelial cells that line the duct normally absorb much of the chloride from the sweat before it hits the skin, leaving sweat only slightly saltier than water.

While Quinton studied the sweat glands, Michael Knowles and Richard Boucher at the University of North Carolina in Chapel Hill looked at the lungs. They found that in people with CF, the epithelial cells lining the airways of the lung also have trouble moving chloride ions across their membranes. Both studies pointed toward a defect that impairs a protein in the cell membrane regulating the flow of chloride ions into and out of epithelial cells.

While these scientists studied the cellular defects behind CF, others were searching for the responsible gene. In 1985, scientists narrowed their search down to chromosome 7. Four years later, they discovered the CFTR gene itself, which lies on chromosome 7. At that time, researchers also identified the ΔF508 mutation that is present on 70 percent of the chromosomes carrying a mutant CFTR gene. They also recognized that a number of other mutations can cause CF, but identified only a few beyond ΔF508. Within eight years, geneticists would identify more than 700 mutations that can cause CF.

In 1990, two groups of researchers working independently presented definitive evidence that tied defects in the CFTR gene with the problems in chloride transport seen in cells from people with CF. One group of researchers, including Lap-Chee Tsui, John Riordan, and Francis Collins (the researchers who discovered the CFTR gene) and their colleagues, showed that they could correct the chloride channel defects in pancreas cells from people with CF by supplying the cells with a copy of the normal CFTR gene. The second group of researchers, led by Michael Welsh and Alan Smith, got the same results using airway epithelial cells taken from people with CF. Again, they found that adding the normal CFTR gene to the defective epithelial cells restored their ability to move chloride ions across cell membranes.

SYMPTOMS OF CF

Understanding the molecular basis of a disease helps scientists to derive new and more effective treatments. But first, parents who suspect their child may have that disease must be able to recognize its symptoms. A child who has been diagnosed with CF early in life can begin to receive the treatments that have been designed to keep people with the disease in good health. The symptoms and their degree of severity vary from person to person. Most people with CF show symptoms by the age of two or three, but those in whom the symptoms are quite mild may go undiagnosed until they are in their teens or twenties. In a few cases, individuals with very mild symptoms may not be diagnosed until they reach middle age.

Although CF presents itself in different ways depending on the age of the affected individual, most people with the disease experience some symptoms as children. The respiratory problems that plague children with CF include chronic *bronchitis* and frequent bouts with *pneumonia*. In addition to lung infections, approximately 85 percent of people with CF experience problems with digestion. They have difficulty digesting food, produce fatty stools, and may "fail to thrive" as children. Children with CF may have ravenous appetites but fail to gain weight despite consuming large quantities of food.

In newborns, the thickened mucus secretions characteristic of CF may cause severe intestinal obstruction, a condition called *meconium ileus*. The waste products present in the intestine of the fetus, called meconium, usually get expelled soon after a child is born. In 5 to 10 percent of children with CF, the meconium does not get excreted, but plugs up the lower portion of the small intestine, called the ileum. The blockage probably occurs because the mucus secreted by the intestines of babies with CF is thicker and more difficult to excrete. Doctors can usually flush the meconium from the intestine using an enema that contains some digestive enzymes to help dissolve the mucous plug.

Sometimes, however, surgery is necessary to remove the blockage. The surgeon removes the area of the ileum where the blockage lies and then sews the two ends of the intestine together again. Because the small intestine is so long—it reaches a length of 20 feet in adults—people can get along fine, digestively speaking, when they're missing a short piece. A person missing a portion of the ileum possesses a somewhat smaller intestinal surface area for absorbing the nutrients from digested food.

Newborns with CF may also appear *jaundiced* after birth, because their *bile ducts* may get clogged with mucus. When bile cannot move from the liver to the intestine—where it helps to digest fat and eliminate certain pigments derived from the breakdown of red blood cells—it is absorbed into the bloodstream. Because bile is greenish in color, an excess of bile pigments in the blood can give the skin a jaundiced, yellow hue.

About 20 percent of children with CF develop *rectal prolapse*, in which part of the rectum protrudes outside the anus. The condition, which may occur because children with CF have bulkier stools due to problems digesting fat, usually disappears when a child receives the proper dietary supplements of pancreatic enzyme. An infant with CF may also experience other symptoms related to poor digestion, including frequent loose stools, a distended abdomen, and poor weight gain despite a healthy appetite. Other early symptoms of CF include recurrent congestion, coughing or wheezing, a salty taste to the sweat, and unexplained dehydration. Because most of these symptoms are not unique to CF and may be somewhat mild, doctors sometimes fail to diagnose the disease in infants.

Older children may suffer from recurrent chest infections and from a susceptibility to heat prostration, whereby they become physically exhausted if they get too hot while playing. Intestinal obstruction can cause a child with CF to be underweight. Some children are not diagnosed with CF until a younger sibling is born with a more severe form of the disease.

The most common symptoms in adolescents or adults include recurrent chest infections, a delayed onset of puberty, and infertility. Approximately 98 percent of adult males with CF are sterile because they lack the *vas deferens*—the tube that carries sperm from the testes. Women with CF may also experience infertility because thickened mucus around the *cervix* may block sperm from fertilizing their eggs. (See chapter 4 for a more detailed description of how CF affects the various organs of the body.)

DIAGNOSING CF

Part of the problem in diagnosing CF lies in the rather common nature of its symptoms. Chest infections can be attributed to chronic bronchitis, pneumonia, or even asthma. And the digestive problems are sometimes mistaken for allergies to foods such as milk or wheat. To diagnose CF, doctors take into account the family's medical history, a physical examination of the child, and the results of tests designed to identify the defects associated with CF.

Physicians have devised a number of different techniques for testing infants, children, or adults for CF. Newborn babies with CF have abnormally high levels of a protein called *immunreactive trypsinogen* (*IRT*) in their blood. Trypsinogen, a protein that is a precursor for the pancreatic enzyme *trypsin*, circulates in the blood and is elevated in newborns with CF. Technicians can measure the levels of IRT from the same dried blood spot they obtain from newborns for other neonatal screening tests. Unfortunately, the IRT test yields a high number of false positives: of every 20 babies who test positive for IRT, only 1 actually has CF. (There is also a low false negative rate.) Coupling the IRT test with genetic testing increases the accuracy of the diagnosis.

To diagnose children with CF, doctors most often turn to the sweat test, which is safe and reliable but must be performed by experienced physicians or hospital staff. The technician places electrodes surrounded by a gauze pad soaked with a drug called pilocarpine on the forearm of the child being tested and wraps the area in plastic. The technician then uses a very weak electric current to drive the pilocarpine into the skin. This harmless drug stimulates the sweat glands to produce sweat. The technician then removes the electrodes and covers the stimulated area with an absorbant piece of filter paper to collect the sweat. After 30 minutes, the technician removes the filter paper and sends it to the laboratory, where the levels of chloride in the child's sweat are measured. Children with CF have levels greater than 60 millimoles (mmol) of salt per liter of sweat (other children have less than 40) and can have 2 to 5 times the normal amount of chloride in their sweat. The test indicates only whether a child has CF. The levels of chloride in the sweat do not correlate with the severity of the disease and cannot be used to predict whether a person will have a mild or severe form of CF.

To diagnose adults suspected of having CF, doctors sometimes measure how well electrical currents can move through the epithelial cells lining the nose. Because these cells rely on the CFTR channel protein to export chloride ions, which generate electrical currents as they move across the cell membrane, doctors can measure abnormal chloride currents in the nasal epithelium of people with CF. This specialized test is performed only in a select few CF centers.

Now that scientists have discovered the CFTR gene and have identified a series of mutations that cause CF, doctors can perform genetic testing to diagnose the disease. To test infants, children, or adults for a mutant CFTR gene, the doctor isolates DNA from a blood sample or a sample of cells scraped from inside the cheek. By analyzing the segment of DNA that carries the CFTR gene, a doctor can tell whether someone has CF or is a carrier. DNA from a carrier of CF would show both normal CFTR sequences and sequences that contain a CFTR mutation.

Fetal DNA can be collected by chorionic villus sampling or by amniocentesis, procedures that will be discussed further in chapter 6.

Although detecting CFTR mutations in a DNA test indicates that a person has CF, a negative result does not necessarily rule out a diagnosis of CF. Because most diagnostic laboratories use tests by which they can identify only a handful of the most common CFTR mutations, DNA testing currently allows physicians to diagnose CF in three-quarters of the people who have the disease. Someone with CF might have an undiscovered CFTR mutation or a mutation for which doctors do not routinely screen patients.

Scientists are currently working toward improving the DNA testing techniques in an effort to make the tests faster and better able to detect a large array of CFTR mutations. One group of scientists working at a California-based biotechnology company called Affymetrix has developed a "DNA chip" that might someday allow doctors to screen for hundreds of different CFTR mutations simultaneously. Each chip contains hundreds, even thousands, of molecular probes designed to detect the deletions and substitutions in CFTR that cause CF. When a DNA sample is applied to the chip, any mutations that match the probes will stick to the chip, allowing scientists to identify them quickly and easily.

PRENATAL AND EARLY SCREENING FOR CF

Because CF is a genetic disorder, people with a family history of the disease may want to screen newborns even before any symptoms arise. Couples who have given birth to a child with CF might also want to test future children prenatally. To do this, doctors remove cells from the *placenta* or from the *amniotic fluid* that surrounds the fetus and test the DNA for CFTR mutations. Again, the same caveats about the accuracy of DNA testing apply to diagnosing unborn children. (See chapter 6 for more details about prenatal diagnosis and family planning for couples who have CF or are carriers.

Does early diagnosis affect the severity of the disease? The results are not clear. Certainly early diagnosis leads to early treatment, which can help alleviate symptoms. Although in 1997 a federal advisory panel recommended that doctors offer genetic testing for CF to couples who are considering having a baby, they did not recommend routine screening of all newborn babies for CF.

3. The Molecular Basis of CF

I believe that the major diseases of human beings have become approachable biological puzzles, ultimately solvable. The great need now, for the medicine of the future, is for more information at the most fundamental levels of the living process.

Lewis Thomas, *A Long Line of Cells*

In hindsight, it seems fairly obvious that a defective ion channel in cell membranes would lie behind the symptoms of CF, from the salty sweat to the thickened mucus. Of course, hindsight is always 20–20. Even if scientists had known for certain that the molecular defect that causes CF is a faulty ion-channel protein, it would not have helped them locate the gene that encodes the CFTR channel. To solve the biological puzzle that is CF, scientists needed to identify the gene responsible and to determine how heritable mutations in that gene precipitate disease. Only then would they be able to develop diagnostic tests for CF and, potentially, more specific and effective treatments.

THE RACE FOR THE GENE

For half a century, scientists have known that CF is a heritable genetic disorder caused by mutations in a single gene. But how do scientists set about finding a gene when they have no idea what it looks like and only an inkling of what it normally does?

For some genetic disorders, the task is made easier because affected individuals have gross chromosomal abnormalities. Certain diseases are caused by huge duplications, deletions, or rearrangements of a person's chromosomal DNA—some large enough for scientists to see when they look at the chromosomes with a microscope. If everyone who has a particular disease also shows a duplication or deletion of a certain hunk of chromosome, scientists know where to begin their search for the responsible gene or genes.

CF, it turns out, is not so simple. Scientists examined the chromosomes of children with CF and found no obvious flaws—no large deletions or rearrangements or breaks. So they suspected that the damage that causes CF must be smaller. Without such defects to guide them, scientists had to figure out the best way to search through all the chromosomes to find the gene responsible for CF. The task was Herculean: human chromosomes contain some 3 billion nucleotide bases, most of which scientists refer to as *junk DNA*. Although junk DNA is not actually trash—it may help to control which genes get turned on in different types of cells—it does not encode genes. So scientists hunting for the CF gene had to work out how to bypass the junk DNA and confine their search to the stretches of DNA that carry genetic information. When one is looking for a needle in a haystack is, the smaller the haystack is, the better.

They turned to a process called *reverse genetics*, which involves identifying a gene by finding the disease-causing mutations that lie within it. The first clue about where to begin the search for mutations came in 1985, when Lap-Chee Tsui and his colleagues at the Toronto Hospital for Sick Children discovered that the gene responsible for CF lies somewhere on human chromosome 7. Their discovery hinged on a technique called *linkage analysis*.

When genes lie near one another on the same chromosome, they tend to be inherited together, like those bestowing red hair and freckles. The closer the genes are on the chromosome, the greater the likelihood is that they will be inherited together.

Scientists located the CF gene by looking for *genetic markers*—distinct bits of DNA sequence—that are frequently inherited by people with CF. The closer the marker sequence lies to the gene that causes CF, the more often it will be inherited along with the defective CF gene in people who have the disease. Once they had located markers that lie very close to the gene that causes CF on chromosome 7, the researchers could begin decoding the sequence of the DNA to look for the actual gene.

For the linkage approach to work, the scientists needed to have access to the DNA from a large numbers of families with CF. In 1986, scientists from almost every major research group searching for the CF gene joined together to pool their data—giving the collaborative group over 200 families in which to search for the marker sequences that would lead them to the gene for CF. And they identified two distinct marker sequences that flanked the putative CF gene. The competition gained momentum: several groups of scientists, in London, Toronto, Salt Lake City, and Boston, set about using these genetic markers to help pin down the CF gene's exact chromosomal address.

But even with markers to guide them, the scientists' search was far from over. Each of these marker sequences sat about 1 million nucleotides away from the putative CF gene—a stretch of DNA that was too large to decode nucleotide by nucleotide. So each group of researchers independently worked on identifying other markers that would bring them closer to the CF gene. In 1989, Dr. Tsui, John Riordan, and their colleagues at the Hospital for Sick Children, and Francis Collins and his colleagues at the University of Michigan in Ann Arbor, identified a candidate gene, which they named CFTR. The researchers had examined approximately 500,000 nucleotides of DNA in the region that contained the CFTR gene. They used a technique they called *chromosome walking*—a process akin to pulling small fistfuls of hay from the haystack and searching each one for the needle. In each handful of DNA the researchers isolated, they looked for certain characteristics that indicate the presence of a gene.

Once they found the CFTR gene, how did the researchers know that it was the gene responsible for CF? They found that in people with CF, the CFTR gene contained mutations that were absent in healthy individuals who did not have CF and who were not CF carriers. And they found that the CFTR gene appeared to encode a protein that could form an ion channel. Further, the researchers determined that the CFTR protein is present largely in epithelial cells—a finding that fit in with what doctors knew about the biology of CF.

More conclusive proof that the CFTR gene was in fact the gene responsible for CF followed in 1990, when researchers showed that adding a normal CFTR gene to airway epithelial cells from a CF patient restored the cells' ability to transport chloride ions. In the same year, Dr. Collins and his colleagues confirmed that CFTR could restore chloride ion transport in epithelial cells taken from the pancreas of a person with CF. These results suggest that someday scientists might be able to treat CF by adding the CFTR gene to the cells that need it, particularly lung epithelial cells. (See chapter 7 for a thorough discussion of the development of CF gene-therapy treatments.)

CFTR: THE GENE, THE PROTEIN

The CFTR gene spans some 230,000 nucleotides, of which about 6,200 encode the actual CFTR protein that forms the ion channels in the cell membrane. The remaining nucleotides form regions of DNA that control which cells produce CFTR channels and when. In complex organisms, genes are laid out in pieces: the *exons*—the bits that encode a protein—are separated by spacer regions of DNA called *introns*. After the molecular machinery in the cell nucleus converts the entire gene into RNA, the introns get snipped out. The 24 CFTR exons, in the form of RNA, then get stitched together to form the messenger RNA that is presented to the cellular machinery that manufactures the CFTR protein (fig. 3.1).

FIG. 3.I. Making CFTR. In the nucleus, specialized molecular machinery converts the CFTR gene into a molecule of messenger RNA. This messenger molecule is shipped out to the endoplasmic reticulum, where another type of cellular machinery produces the CFTR protein. The protein makes its way through the cytoplasm (via complex pathways not shown here) and is inserted into the cell membrane, where it can function as an ion channel that allows chloride to pass into and out of the cell.

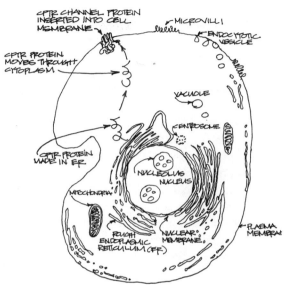

FIG. 3.2. The CFTR channel. In this schematic cartoon, chloride ions pass out of a cell through the pore formed by the membrane-spanning segments of the CFTR protein. The nucleotide-binding domains cleave the high-energy bonds of a molecule called ATP, perhaps providing the energy needed to pump chloride ions through the channel. The regulatory domain may control the function of the CFTR channel.

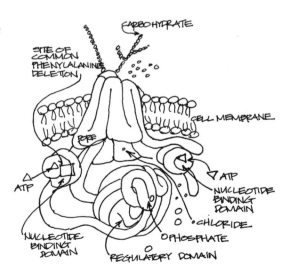

The CFTR protein contains five main structural regions or *domains* (fig. 3.2). Two of the domains penetrate through the cell membrane, forming the pore through which chloride ions pass. Another two regions dwell in the cell cytoplasm, where they bind *ATP*—an energy-rich molecule that powers many cellular reactions. By cleaving the high-energy bonds in the ATP molecules, these domains might open the channel and allow chloride ions to pass through. Finally, a large *regulatory domain* may control the activity of the CFTR channel. This domain contains sites that can be *phosphorylated*—a chemical modification that may help to promote the passage of chloride ions through the pore. Although researchers have some idea about what the CFTR protein may look like, they are far from knowing exactly how it works. Many researchers argue about whether the CFTR protein can transport ATP into and out of the cell. Others are investigating whether the CFTR protein might influence the activity of other chloride channels or sodium channels in epithelial cells.

The CFTR protein is not exactly unique. The channel resembles other proteins that belong to a large family called the *ABC proteins*—molecules that all contain an *ATP binding cassette*. Over the past several years, scientists have identified more than 100 genes that encode ABC proteins. One of the most infamous, the *multidrug resistance protein*, renders human cancer cells resistant to a variety of chemotherapeutic agents by enabling them to pump out the toxic drugs. By studying how other ABC proteins function, scientists may learn more about CFTR.

THE MUTATIONS THAT CAUSE CF

Any one of more than 700 different mutations in the CFTR gene can cause CF. The most common mutation, ΔF508, prevents the CFTR channel from reaching the cell membrane (fig 3.3, class II mutations). Instead, the protein gets trapped in the

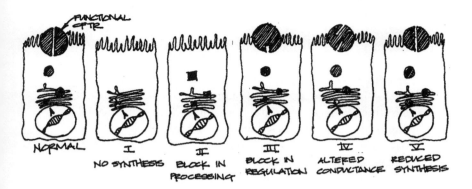

FIG. 3.3. CFTR mutations. Mutations in the CFTR gene can cause CF in different ways. Some prevent the synthesis of the CFTR channel altogether (class I). Others direct the production of a channel that never makes it to the cell membrane (class II), a channel that fails to respond to regulatory signals in the cell (class III), or a channel that doesn't move chloride ions as efficiently as normal CFTR channels do (class IV). Finally, some mutations may affect how much CFTR protein is made by the cell (class V).

endoplasmic reticulum—the cellular compartment that serves as a birthing chamber for new proteins. Some researchers have found that forcing the ΔF508 CFTR channel to insert into the cell membrane restores some of the cell's ability to transport chloride ions. If scientists can figure out how to coax ΔF508 into cell membranes in patients, they might be well on their way to curing a majority of people with CF.

Other mutations in the CFTR gene amount to premature stop signals that place a period before the end of the CFTR sentence. When the molecular machinery that makes proteins encounters this stop signal, it abandons work on CFTR, producing a protein that's only a fraction of its normal size. These aborted CFTR protein fragments are destroyed by the cell. So people with CF who have the premature stop type of mutation in their CFTR genes wind up with no CFTR protein at all (fig. 3.3, class I mutations).

In many cases, changing only a single nucleotide base can generate a premature stop signal in the CFTR gene sequence. For example, the second most common mutation in CF—designated G542X—changes a glycine (G) amino-acid residue at position 542 in the CFTR protein into a premature stop signal (X). The string of three nucleotides that codes for glycine is GGA, but TGA is one of the stop signals that tells the cell machinery when it has finished synthesizing the whole protein. So changing the first G to a T in the CFTR gene signals the cell machinery that its job is done before it actually makes a full-sized CFTR protein. The truncated CFTR protein cannot function and gets destroyed in the cell cytoplasm, leaving the cell with few, if any, functional CFTR channels in the cell membrane.

A third class of mutation generates a dysfunctional CFTR protein that is normal in size but contains an incorrect amino acid somewhere along its length. For example, the third most common CFTR mutation, called G551D, codes for a protein that has an aspartic acid (D) at position 551 in the protein chain, rather than the normal glycine (G). Again, this mutation results from a change in a single nucleotide base in the CFTR gene. The nucleotide triplet GGT codes for the amino acid glycine, and GAT codes for aspartic acid. So changing the middle G to an A in the CFTR gene will instruct the molecular machinery that makes the protein to insert an aspartic acid rather than a glycine residue in the CFTR channel. A CFTR protein sporting this substitution can insert into the cell membrane correctly but does not respond properly to the chemical cues that help to control its function.

Some mutations cause the cell to make CFTR proteins that are lazy. These mutant channels allow chloride ions to pass into or out of the cell but do not work as hard as normal CFTR channels to maintain the proper salt balance (fig. 3.3, class IV).

Such mutations might impair ion transport by introducing a flaw into the lining of the pore of the CFTR channel.

Finally, other substitutions do not affect CFTR function at all, but they impair how much of the protein is made by the cell (fig. 3.3, class V). Some of these mutations fall in the junctions between the intron and exon sequences in the CFTR gene, preventing the cellular machinery from correctly excising an intron. In people with CF who have this type of mutation, few functional channels reach the cell membrane.

CFTR mutations occur at different frequencies in different racial groups. For example, although the mutation G542X accounts for only about 2.5 percent of the CF mutations worldwide, it is found in 8 percent of people with CF in Spain and Mexico and 13 percent of Ashkenazi Jews with CF. The mutation M1101K (substitution of a lysine residue for a methionine at position 1101) accounts for 69 percent of CF cases in the Hutterite population in Canada. And in a small study of the Zuni Native Americans of New Mexico, the mutation R1162X (replacing an arginine with a stop code at position 1162) has been detected in every individual with CF. To keep up with the ever-increasing number of CF mutations scientists are discovering, Dr. Tsui and his colleagues have formed the CF Genetic Analysis Consortium, which maintains a database of information on the genetic defects that cause CF. (See appendix A for more information about this electronic database.)

ANIMAL STUDIES

Much of what scientists know about how the CFTR protein functions—and how mutations can shut it down—comes from studies of the CFTR ion channel in animal cells. Some researchers examine how the natural CFTR channels made in the lung epithelial cells of animals—including dogs, rats, sheep, and rhesus monkeys—transport chloride ions. Others introduce the human CFTR gene into animal cells that can be maintained easily in the laboratory. Such studies can reveal how the gene directs the production of a human CFTR protein, how the protein works, and how mutations disrupt its function. Animals, particularly rats and monkeys, also provide a means by which scientists can evaluate CF gene therapy methods for safety and efficiency before testing them in humans.

At first glance, it might seem a waste of time to study the CFTR proteins from animals when scientists can study human CFTR directly. But animal cells are often easier to manipulate in the laboratory, and animal CFTR genes and proteins can be remarkably similar to their human counterparts. In fact, to determine which parts of the human CFTR protein are most important for its proper function, scientists have compared the sequences of CFTR genes from a variety of mammals, including mice, monkeys, humans, cows, sheep, and pigs. Because evolutionary forces tend to favor things that work, the regions of a protein that are critical for its function—and the portions of the gene that encode them—are often conserved from species to species. For example, scientists find that the sequence of exon II in the CFTR gene, a region targeted by a number of mutations that cause severe cases of CF in humans, is highly conserved among different mammals. The regions of the CFTR gene that encode the portions of the ion channel that anchor CFTR in the cell membrane are also highly conserved, suggesting that these regions are important for chloride transport.

Scientists also use animal cells as a sort of living test tube in which to study the human CFTR channel. For example, researchers can inject frog eggs with the human CFTR gene and coax them into producing a human CFTR protein. Using this system, scientists can study a variety of mutant CFTR proteins and determine which amino-acid residues are important for chloride-ion transport and how mutations affect the production and processing of the CFTR protein. Scientists first discovered that the $\Delta F508$ mutant CFTR channel never gets to its proper place in the cell membrane, in part, by studying the production of the protein in cells derived from the kidneys of monkeys.

Further, scientists studying the processing of human ΔF508 mutant CFTR protein in animal cells found that when they lowered the temperature of the cells making the mutant CFTR, the channel protein gets into the cell membrane and transports chloride ions almost as well as normal CFTR. Although scientists cannot treat people with CF by lowering the temperature of their lung cells, the study suggests that if the ΔF508 mutant CFTR protein can somehow be escorted to the cell membrane it might function well enough to effectively cure the disease.

Rhesus monkeys are the animals of choice for researchers who wish to test new gene-therapy strategies. Before using a virus to deliver a normal CFTR gene to the lung epithelial cells of CF patients in clinical trials, researchers tested it first in monkeys. Unfortunately, monkeys also make their own CFTR protein. So scientists studying gene-therapy protocols in monkeys can only determine whether a virus delivers the gene to the lungs; they cannot examine whether the human CFTR proteins function properly.

Ultimately, scientists would like to develop an animal model of CF—an animal, lacking a functional CFTR ion channel, which displays symptoms similar to the ones experienced by humans with the disease. To that end, several groups of scientists in 1992 generated mouse models of CF. These CFTR-deficient mice, like humans with CF, displayed defects in the transport of chloride ions in their airway and intestinal epithelial cells. They also experienced intestinal problems similar to meconium ileus in humans.

Unfortunately, because many of the mice lacking CFTR die of intestinal blockage soon after birth and do not survive long enough to develop the lung problems that most often prove fatal in people with CF, a study of respiratory problems in this model is not feasible. When the mice do survive, they do not appear to develop any respiratory disease. Perhaps the CFTR-deficient mice produce an alternate chloride channel in their lung cells but not in their intestinal epithelium. Scientists might use these mice to learn how to trick the lung epithelial cells in people with

CF into manufacturing an alternative chloride ion channel that might compensate for their defective CFTR. The mice might also lead to the discovery of other genes that influence the severity of CF in humans. Dr. Tsui has found that other genetic factors might influence the progression of the disease in CFTR-deficient mice.

Because mice are small and relatively short-lived, they might not prove to be the best model for studying CF. People with CF experience lung infections that lead to chronic respiratory problems over a period of years. Some scientists are turning to livestock—in particular, sheep—for a better model of human CF. Such large animals might be able to develop lung problems that more closely mimic the symptoms of CF in humans. Some scientists are trying to develop techniques for deleting or disrupting the CFTR gene in sheep. Others are searching for sheep that have natural mutations in their CFTR genes. If researchers succeed in identifying CFTR mutants in sheep, they should be able to breed animals that show symptoms typical of CF in humans. Such an animal model would also provide scientists with a better system for testing potential CF treatments. (See chapter 7 for a review of the experimental therapies that scientists are developing to treat CF.)

4. How CF Affects the Body

We have today an impressive mastery of our illnesses precisely because we have a systematic insight into the processes which constitute health.

Jonathan Miller, M.D., *The Body in Question*

Understanding the biology of human disease depends on understanding how the body functions normally. To appreciate how CF disrupts the activity of the lungs, the pancreas, and other organs, we need to know how the systems affected by CF work in a healthy individual. Although persistent bronchial infections and progressive lung deterioration present the most serious health problems for people with CF, the disease affects a number of organ systems in the body, particularly the exocrine glands (fig. 4.1). Unlike the *endocrine glands* (such as the pituitary, thyroid, and adrenal glands), which secrete their hormones directly into the bloodstream, the exocrine glands dump their enzymes and metabolites into ducts that lead out of the body or into hollow organs, such as the intestine. This chapter examines the major systems damaged by CF—the lungs and respiratory system, the pancreas and digestive system, the sweat glands, and the reproductive tracts. We'll see how these systems function normally and how CF impairs that activity.

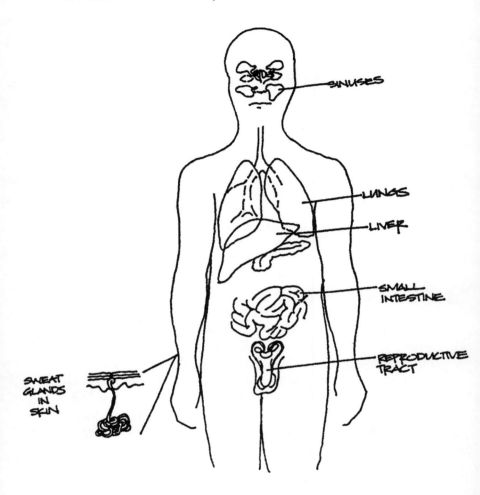

FIG. 4.1. Organs affected by CF. Although the deterioration of lung function presents the most serious health problems for people with CF, the disease affects a number of organ systems in the body, including the pancreas, sweat glands, reproductive tract, intestines, liver, and sinuses.

THE LUNGS AND THE RESPIRATORY SYSTEM

The respiratory system brings *oxygen* into the body and expels *carbon dioxide*. Cells all over the body require oxygen to produce energy. The body can last only a few minutes without oxygen before irreversible damage occurs. In the lungs, blood exchanges oxygen for carbon dioxide. Red blood cells ferry oxygen to all the tissues of the body and carry away carbon dioxide. The respiratory system also filters, warms, and humidifies inhaled air so the lungs can perform optimally.

The anatomy of the lung makes this spongy organ well suited to its task. Its air passages resemble a tree, dividing into finer and finer branches and terminating in tiny sacs that exchange gases with the blood coming from and returning to the heart (fig. 4.2). Inhaled air enters through the nose and mouth and sweeps down the *trachea*, a muscular tube surrounded by rings of cartilage that protect it and prevent it from collapsing during breathing. About halfway down the breastbone, the trachea divides into the two main or *primary bronchi* that shunt air to the right and left lungs. Like a branching tree, the primary bronchi divide again into five *secondary bronchi* that supply air to the five *lobes* of the lung—three in the right lung and two in the left. The bronchi continue to divide into smaller and smaller passageways. As the airways become smaller, they become thinner and less muscular.

Eventually the smallest *bronchioles* dead-end in tiny, thin-walled sacs called *alveoli*. The lungs contain about 300 million of these sacs, which look like little bunches of grapes. They inflate and deflate like tiny balloons with every breath. The all-important gas exchange occurs in these delicate clusters of alveoli. The walls of the alveoli are only one cell-layer thick and each little sac is nestled snugly into a bed of *capillaries* that receive the oxygen-poor blood delivered by the circulatory system. Oxygen from inhaled air simply diffuses through the wall of the alveolus and across the wall of the capillary—also one

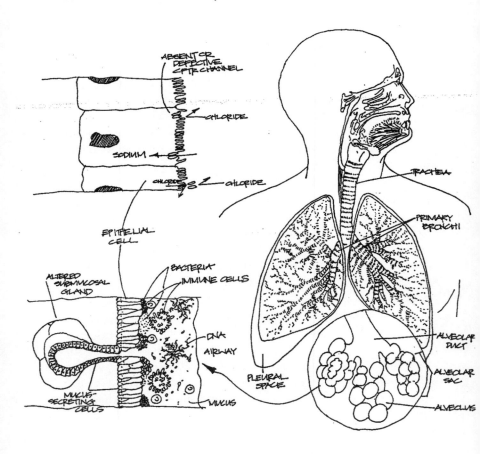

FIG. 4.2. CF and the lung. The major airways of the lungs divide into finer and finer branches, finally terminating in tiny sacs called alveoli that exchange oxygen and carbon dioxide with the blood in neighboring capillaries. When the CFTR channels in the epithelial cells that line the respiratory tract are defective, salt accumulates in the mucus that helps trap particles and bacteria so that they can be removed from the lungs. The salty mucus present in the lungs of CF patients is thick and difficult to expel. DNA released from bacteria and invading immune cells makes the mucus stickier still.

cell thick—and into the bloodstream. At the same time, carbon dioxide passes from the bloodstream into the alveolus where it waits to be exhaled. In the exchange, red blood cells give up the carbon dioxide and accept the oxygen, transporting it back to the heart so it can be delivered to the rest of the body.

How does CF impair respiration? Mostly by clogging the airways with mucus. The entire respiratory system is lined with epithelial cells, and interspersed between these cells are mucous glands. They secrete a thin layer of mucus that coats the inside of the passages, facilitating the movement of gases through the thin alveolar walls, keeping the airway membranes moist, and helping to clear particles and microbes from the lungs. When the mucus traps particles and bacteria, they are then swept along by the *cilia*—little hairlike projections that fringe the epithelial cells and beat in a single direction—up and out of the lungs. Although many airborne particles are filtered out by the nose and never reach the lungs, it's up to the mucus and cilia to trap and push any particles and bacteria that reach the lower respiratory tract up into the bronchi, where they can be expelled from the lungs by a sneeze or a cough or a swallow.

The defect in the CFTR channel causes the mucus in the lungs to be thicker and stickier than normal. Because the thicker mucus does not flow as easily, it tends to block the smaller airways. With the smaller airways plugged by mucus, the lungs lose some of their capacity, preventing adequate exchange of oxygen and carbon dioxide. In general terms, this loss of lung function is labeled as *chronic obstructive pulmonary disease*, the most serious problem in people with CF. Airways and alveoli that are cut off from the rest of the lung often collapse and form scar tissue. For the person with CF, this airway obstruction causes distress—coughing, wheezing, and an increased susceptibility to lung infections.

The obstruction starts in the smaller airways. A condition called *bronchiolitis* results when the bronchioles become plugged by mucus and inflamed. Eventually, infections develop and the larger tubes become inflamed, leading to chronic *bronchitis*.

Chronic infections and obstruction can cause the bronchial walls to balloon and weaken, a condition called *bronchiectasis*.

People with CF can also get *emphysema*, a disease in which alveoli and the small air passages become overdistended because air trapped inside them cannot escape. Emphysema also weakens the elasticity of the lungs. If the distended alveoli rupture, a person with CF could develop *pneumothorax,* a condition in which a tear in the lung tissue allows air to get trapped in the space outside the lung. As more air escapes into the chest cavity, the damaged lung can collapse.

Interestingly, the lungs of people with CF look normal at birth. This suggests that as a person with CF gets older, the recurring cycles of infection and inflammation progressively damage the lungs.

The thickened mucus that builds up in the lungs of people with CF also encourages chest infections by making it more difficult for the respiratory system to clear particles and microbes. The cycle is made worse because the infections themselves further inflame the airways and prompt the lungs to generate even more mucus. When the microbes get mired in the thick mucus, the lungs respond by trying to wash the bacteria away with more mucus. *Neutrophils*—the white blood cells that fight infections—also rush in to engulf the microbes and themselves become trapped by the thick mucus. People with CF often have 1,000 times the number of dead white blood cells in their lungs than people without the disease. The trapped neutrophils eventually burst open and spill long, sticky strands of their DNA into the mucus, further increasing its viscosity and worsening the infection.

The common bacterium *Staphylococcus aureus* usually causes the earliest lung infections in people with CF. By age 10, most children with CF have already been infected by *S. aureus*. Later in the course of the disease, the lungs become colonized by *Pseudomonas aeruginosa*, a microbe that attacks damaged tissue. Some people with CF also fall prey to infections with various fungi, such as *Aspergillus*.

Failure to clear these infections can lead to respiratory failure, in which the lungs are no longer able to keep the body supplied with oxygen and free of excess carbon dioxide. With less oxygen in the blood, the heart may also try to work harder to circulate an increased volume of blood through the lungs. The resulting increase in blood pressure could cause the right ventricle of the heart to thicken and enlarge. This added strain of pumping blood through the lungs can damage the heart muscle. The obstruction of the lungs with mucus can be kept to a minimum with daily physiotherapy and the chest infections held at bay with the proper antibiotics. (See chapter 5 for a detailed discussion of these and other respiratory treatments.)

The development of lung disease also causes in nearly all people with CF a somewhat curious condition called *clubbing*, which is an enlargement or rounding of the tips of the fingers and toes. It appears that substances released in response to lung infections enter the bloodstream and somehow stimulate the growth of the soft tissue at the base of the fingernails and toenails.

People with CF also develop *sinusitis*, an inflammation of the sinus cavities in the head, and many experience the growth of *polyps* in their nasal passages, perhaps also due to the thick mucus that causes congestion of the membranes lining these passages.

THE PANCREAS AND THE DIGESTIVE SYSTEM

The human digestive system is basically one long tube with a lot of specialized parts, designed to process food. From the mouth through to the intestines, the digestive system breaks down ingested food, mechanically and chemically, into the molecules that provide the raw materials used by cells to fulfill their basic metabolic needs. With the help of enzymes secreted by organs including the pancreas, the gut reduces proteins to amino acids, carbohydrates to simple sugars, and fats to glycerol and fatty acids. Cells throughout the body then use the amino acids for tissue growth and repair and for synthesizing needed proteins, including enzymes. Sugars and glycerol provide the body with sources of energy. Fatty acids aid in the absorption of some vitamins and get incorporated into cell membranes. The small intestine performs the bulk of the work in extracting and absorbing the usable nutrients derived from the digestion of food. Indigestible materials are excreted as wastes.

Digestion begins in the mouth. The *salivary glands* secrete an enzyme called *amylase*, which begins the process of digesting starches. Chewing food mechanically reduces it to smaller, more easily digestible pieces and mixes it with the amylase in the saliva. Swallowed food goes to the stomach, where it is attacked by the *hydrochloric acid* and *pepsin* secreted by specialized cells lining the stomach. As the stomach churns, the pepsin reduces proteins into smaller molecules called peptides. The partially digested food then passes into the small intestine.

Most of the digestion and absorption takes place in the small intestine. And that's where the pancreas comes in. An organ the size and shape of a large dog's tongue, the adult human pancreas is about 6 inches long and weighs about 3 ounces. When food leaves the stomach, the pancreas and the liver secrete digestive juices into the small intestine to complete the digestive process. The liver provides bile, which helps to emulsify fats. The pancreas supplies a handful of enzymes critical for the complete digestion of a meal: *trypsin* and *chymotrypsin* reduce proteins and peptides to their constituent amino acids, *lipase* breaks down emulsified fats to glycerol and fatty acids, and a bit more amylase turns any remaining starches into disaccharides. Altogether, the pancreas can synthesize and secrete about 2 pints of digestive enzymes per day—that's 32 ounces of product from a 3-ounce organ.

The intestine also secretes enzymes of its own to break down peptides and to reduce disaccharides to glucose, the main source of energy for cells. These nutrients are absorbed by the *microvilli*—the fingerlike projections that cover the folded inner surface of the small intestine. Each microvillus is surrounded by capillaries carrying the blood that takes up the digested nutrients and transports them to the cells of the body.

Inside the pancreas, cells called *acini* synthesize the digestive enzymes. These cells lie in little clusters that surround tiny ducts, like the stones that surround a well. The acinar cells secrete enzymes into the small central duct, which connects with larger and larger ducts, like small roads merging into larger streets and eventually into the highway. Pancreatic enzymes and the bile from the liver flow into a large common duct before they enter the small intestine.

In the majority of people with CF, thick mucus can block the ducts in the pancreas, particularly the smaller ones. The mucous plugs, combined with the backup of enzymes in the pancreas, cause the formation of cysts and eventually scar tissue. As a result, pancreatic enzymes do not reach the small intestine, causing proteins and fats to leave the body as undigested waste. Unless a person with CF takes enzyme supplements, this poor utilization of nutrients can lead to malnourishment, even when the individual consumes more than adequate amounts of food. About 85 percent of people with CF experience pancreatic problems, or *pancreatic insufficiency*. The obstruction—and destruction—of the pancreas usually begins before birth and gradually worsens with time. People with CF usually take pancreatic enzyme supplements with their meals to replace the natural enzymes that never make it to the small intestine. (See chapter 5 for a discussion of nutritional treatments for people with CF.)

A small percentage of adolescents and adults with CF also develop *diabetes*. In addition to the acinar cells producing digestive enzymes, the pancreas also contains cells that secrete *insulin* into the bloodstream. This critical hormone lowers the levels of sugar in the blood. In most diabetics, the insulin-secreting *beta* cells in the pancreas degenerate. In people with CF, the mucous plugs or the fibrous scar tissue in the pancreas probably impinge on the small islands of beta cells, preventing them from secreting insulin and ultimately destroying them. Diabetes does not usually appear until a person with CF reaches adolescence, and the condition can be controlled with insulin.

About 5 to 10 percent of people with CF experience liver dysfunction. Again, ducts in the liver become clogged with mucus, and the condition can lead to *cirrhosis*, in which fibrous scar tissue forms. Why some people with CF develop liver problems and others do not remains unclear.

SWEAT GLANDS

The *sweat glands* help to regulate body temperature, and they also excrete some wastes, such as excess salt and small amounts of *urea*. Humans possess some 2 million sweat glands, each a tightly coiled tube buried in the epidermis, the skin's outermost layer. With each coiled duct measuring about 50 inches in length, that comes out to 6 miles of sweat duct per person.

Sweat contains a dilute solution of chemical *electrolytes*— mostly sodium and chloride, with smaller amounts of calcium and potassium. The sweat from people with CF can contain 5 times the normal amounts of sodium chloride, hence its excessively salty taste. The body produces anywhere from 1 pint to half a gallon of sweat per day. As sweat evaporates from the skin, it helps to cool the body.

Though the sweat ducts of people with CF appear to be physically normal, their ability to reabsorb sodium chloride is impaired. Normally, sweat pools in the base of the gland and then moves through the duct toward the surface of the skin. As sweat flows up and out of the body, channels that line the duct reabsorb the salt ions. CF impairs the ability of the sweat glands to reclaim chloride ions, a defect that may relate directly to the malfunctioning of the CFTR channel that is defective in people with CF. (The functioning of the CFTR chloride ion channel is described in greater detail in chapters 1 and 3.)

Although excreting excess salt in the sweat is generally not a life-threatening condition, excessive loss of electrolytes can become dangerous in hot weather or when a person with CF engages in heavy exercise or runs a fever. People with CF can become dehydrated faster or experience heat stroke more readily than healthy individuals. Because of the salt imbalance, people with CF should drink electrolyte solutions or eat salty foods, especially when they have a fever or exercise strenuously.

REPRODUCTIVE SYSTEMS

The difficulties with the male and female reproductive systems in people with CF also stem from the obstruction of important ducts and passageways by thickened mucous secretions. CF causes infertility in men more often than in women.

About 98 percent of men with CF are infertile. In such men, the epididymis and the vas deferens end in blind alleys or are missing altogether. These tubes normally carry sperm from the testes to the *prostate gland*, where they mix with the other components of *semen*. The vas deferens is the tube that physicians sever during a vasectomy; in essence, males with CF receive a biological vasectomy before birth. Infertile men with CF still manufacture sperm, but the sperm never make it into the ejaculate.

Men with CF undergo normal sexual growth and development, although their sexual maturation may begin later or proceed more slowly than in healthy men. The respiratory difficulties and nutritional deficits experienced by people with CF generally tax their bodies' energy reserves and can sometimes slow their development. Men with CF have a normal sex drive and are capable of normal sexual performance, but the majority cannot father children. Men with CF, however, should not assume they are infertile. To determine their fertility, sexually mature men with CF can ask their doctors to perform a sperm count on their semen.

Most men with CF are born without vas deferens entirely—a condition referred to as *congenital bilateral absence of the vas deferens* (CBAVD). In the late 1960s, scientists realized that this defect was probably caused by the degeneration of the obstructed vas deferens in the fetus. CBAVD sometimes occurs in men without CF; about 80 percent of men with CBAVD harbor at least one mutation in the CFTR gene.

Infertility is not as prevalent in women with CF. In the reproductive tract of a woman with CF, however, the thickened mucus that surrounds the cervix may provide a biological barrier that blocks sperm from passing through the *vagina* and into the *uterus*. Thus a woman with CF may be unable to conceive because sperm cells never make it to her *fallopian tubes*, where they would normally meet and fertilize an ovum.

Women with CF also undergo normal sexual growth and development, although, again, their sexual maturation may begin later or proceed more slowly than in healthy women. Women with CF also lead normal sex lives, and most can become pregnant, but they should carefully consider the risks before deciding to have children. Probably because of their respiratory difficulties, women with CF tend to have higher rates of spontaneous abortions, premature deliveries, and stillbirths.

5. Current Treatments and Health Care Issues

By the year 2000, nearly half of all patients with CF will be adults.

Bonnie Ramsey, M.D.,
University of Washington School of Medicine

As treatments continue to improve, people with CF are living longer and healthier lives. Now that the disease can be managed, children with CF miss less school, and adults with CF can lead fuller, more active lives. This chapter reviews the current treatments available and discusses how people with CF can get the most from their health care providers.

Adults with CF pretty much become their own doctors and health care advocates as they learn to administer treatments, assess their condition, and get the most out of the health care system, particularly with the rise of health maintenance organizations and other managed care plans. Many people with CF choose to visit a CF clinic in addition to seeing their general physician. (See appendix D for listing of CF centers around the country.) The professionals at these centers—pediatricians, dietitians, pulmonary function specialists, psychologists, and social workers—specialize in treating people with CF. Because a body of expert knowledge has been accumulated at such clinics, people with CF and the parents of children with CF can feel that they are receiving the most advanced treatments and advice. The clinics also provide opportunities for people with

CF to participate in research projects and to meet others with the disease.

Most visits to these clinics include a thorough physical exam. Doctors record the patient's weight and height and usually measure lung function. If the person shows any sign of infection, the doctor will take a throat swab or sputum sample to determine what type of bacteria might be present in the lung.

Current treatments are aimed at helping people with CF alleviate their symptoms so they can lead relatively normal lives, enjoying school, work, family, and friends. In general, treatments address problems of breathing and of digestion. Enzyme supplements, taken with meals and snacks, aid people with CF in digesting their food. Daily physiotherapy and exercise help to keep their lungs clear and to build cardiovascular fitness. Antibiotics give some relief from lung infections. When these treatments no longer improve lung function, a person with CF may consider having a lung transplant.

EXERCISE

Physicians consider exercise one of the most beneficial "proactive" treatments for people with CF. In addition to keeping the lungs clear of mucus and building strength and endurance, exercise can give people with CF a sense of well-being and independence. Aerobic exercise, in particular, allows people with CF to move a large volume of air through their lungs, helping to break up mucus and prevent airways from becoming blocked. Aerobics train the body to use oxygen more efficiently and help to preserve the elasticity of the lung walls, which enables the lungs to better disperse mucus. Bacteria generally prefer to colonize moist areas that do not experience a great deal of air flow, so exercise helps to make the lung environment a less hospitable place for microbes.

What constitutes the best type of exercise depends on the person—physicians encourage people with CF to choose exercises that they enjoy. Daily aerobics, including swimming, biking, running, and bouncing on a trampoline, help to strengthen the breathing muscles and build cardiovascular fitness. Nonaerobic exercises, such as weight lifting, are also useful, contributing to an increase of muscle mass and body weight. People with CF can also participate in various sports—basketball, tennis, softball, or just about anything they enjoy. In addition to building strength, physical activity helps to loosen the mucus in the lungs and to stimulate coughing, which helps clear the mucus.

PHYSIOTHERAPY AND RESPIRATORY TREATMENTS

The most serious problems in people with CF are respiratory; therefore, most treatments center on keeping the lungs clear and bringing infections under control. Treatments include the chemical and physical dislodging and removal of mucus from the lungs and the use of antibiotics to manage bacterial infections. In addition to listening to the lungs through a stethoscope and recording patients' descriptions of their symptoms, physicians use lung function tests, X-rays, and other chest scans to help diagnose the condition of the lungs. Symptoms of infection flare-ups or worsening of lung function can include increased coughing or wheezing, increased fatigue and decreased ability to exercise, formation of a barrel-shaped chest due to trapped air in the lungs, weight loss, poor appetite, and fever.

Tests: X-rays, chest scans, and lung function

Yearly chest X-rays can provide information about how CF is affecting the lungs. An X-ray allows a doctor to examine the general shape of the lungs in the chest cavity and to detect areas that appear to be either over-distended with trapped air or damaged so that less air than normal is being received.

Chest scans are less commonly used in the clinic. For this procedure, the person with CF inhales radioactive particles into the lungs. These harmless particles penetrate the air spaces in the lungs, and doctors examine the resulting scan to see if any areas of the lung appear to be receiving too little air. When similarly radioactive substances are injected into a person's bloodstream, the doctor can look to see whether the blood supply to the lungs is even. Chest scans can reveal damage to areas of the lung that might not be detectable by X-ray or stethoscope. When doctors detect an area of the lung that is poorly ventilated or has inadequate blood supply, they can target the specific region with more aggressive physiotherapy to help clear it. Although rarely used in the clinic, chest scans often help scientists involved in clinical trials determine whether experimental drugs are effective in helping patients with CF clear particles and microbes from their lungs.

Lung function tests measure lung volume and how rapidly a person can move air into and out of the lungs. Physicians use the lung function test to keep track of a patient's lung volume over time and to detect *bronchospasm*—a tightening of the airways that makes breathing difficult for asthmatics and people with CF. The test involves inhaling deeply and then exhaling rapidly into a tube connected to a machine called a spirometer, which records the amount of air exhaled. People with CF who experience bronchospasms can take *bronchodilators* to relieve the constriction. Doctors also sometimes prescribe inhaled *steroids* to treat or prevent lung inflammation.

Clearing mucus: physiotherapy and DNase

Daily *chest physiotherapy* (*CPT*) involves thumping on the chest and back of a person with CF to help dislodge and expel the thick mucus from the lungs. This is combined with *bronchial* or *postural draining*, in which the person lies in various positions (or postures) to permit gravity to help the mucus drain toward the throat, where it can be coughed up most easily. Different positions help drain different portions of the lung.

In most cases, the parent performs CPT on a child with CF. In a typical physiotherapy session, the parent positions the child to allow a particular region of the lung to drain, then claps or thumps that portion of the chest to help dislodge the mucus and stimulate its movement. The thumping or percussion should last a few minutes in a particular area, with the child then coughing up and swallowing the mucus. Percussion should be vigorous and rhythmic but not painful. Parents should cup their hands to trap a cushion of air between the palm and the chest, which softens the clapping. The child should wear loose comfortable clothing for a CPT session. Parents should not thump the child on his or her bare skin.

Figure 5.1 shows a few positions for draining different lobes of the lung. Parents should center the percussion over the ribs and avoid thumping the spine, breastbone, stomach, or back to minimize trauma to the spleen, liver, or kidneys. For some reason, the upper lobes of the lungs are particularly prone to bacterial infection; these areas may require extra physiotherapy.

Although parental percussion is the best way to clear mucus in young children with CF, older children can play a more active role in their physiotherapy treatments by performing breathing exercises to develop their respiratory muscles. Breathing exercises involve alternating periods of ordinary breathing with chest expansion—breathing in as deeply as possible from the belly and then exhaling normally. During physiotherapy, the person with CF should also engage in rapid, forced exhalation called *huffing*. Huffing might even be more effective than coughing for clearing mucus from the lungs. This forced exhalation also helps the person gauge how much mucus is left in the lung. Rough, rattly huffing indicates that mucus still remains.

Parents, grandparents, and older siblings of children with CF can help with the physiotherapy at home. People with CF usually receive chest physiotherapy twice a day, often in the mornings and the evenings, when it is least disruptive of everyone's work and school schedules. To help keep their lungs clear and well exercised, people with CF should receive physiotherapy regularly, not just when they have a cough or congestion, although additional sessions may be needed when a child is

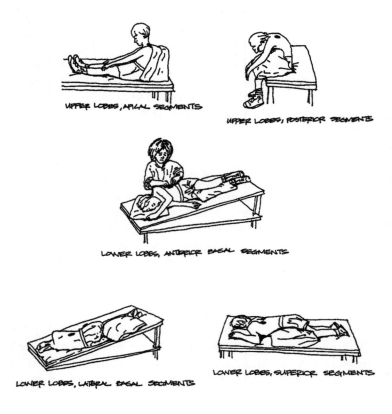

FIG. 5.I. Chest physiotherapy. Some common positions for bronchial drainage. The center panel shows where a parent should thump to help clear mucus from an area in the lower lobes of the lungs. Four other panels show positions for clearing other regions of the lung. The dark ovals indicate where the parent or therapist should concentrate the percussion.

congested. Parents should avoid performing physiotherapy right after mealtimes so the child does not vomit. Each session takes about half an hour.

Morning physiotherapy is important for clearing mucus that builds up overnight. If the person with CF is suffering a bronchospasm, using a bronchodilator inhaler before CPT can help make breathing easier. Aerosolized antibiotics should always be taken after physiotherapy, when the medication can best penetrate the newly cleared lungs and can remain there until the next session.

Physiotherapy need not be a chore, and many parents use CPT as a chance to spend some time with their children, scheduling the session during a favorite TV show or using the time to play a tape or tell stories. To amuse young children, parents can invent blowing or coughing games, or the child can roll around on a *physioball*, which is about 3 feet in diameter. Percussion can be more effective with a physioball, because vibrations bounce through the ball and rebound back to the chest from the opposite side. Children enjoy playing with the ball, and parents find it easier to move the child around to find the best positions for mucus drainage.

Adolescents and adults with CF can learn to perform CPT on themselves, using various types of mechanical percussors or chest clappers to help dislodge the mucus. One such product, called the *Flimm fighter*, comes equipped with three different physiotherapy attachments. Another aide, called a *flutter*, is a small pipe with a marble in it. When a person with CF blows into the pipe, the marble flutters, sending a vibration down the airways to help loosen mucus. Physicians at any CF clinic can help direct people to places where they can purchase such equipment, including an adjustable table for postural drainage.

Parents of children with CF need to remember that coughing is normal and should not be suppressed; it is a natural way for the lungs to clear themselves of debris and mucus. Parents may have to remind others that CF is not contagious, and that children with CF cannot transmit the disease with their coughing.

In 1994, the Food and Drug Administration approved a drug called *DNase* for treatment of people with CF. This aerosolized enzyme breaks down the sticky strands of DNA that spill out of cells that are killed as a result of chronic airway infections: bacteria, neutrophils, and the infected epithelial cells themselves. The drug may help people who have a moderate case of CF and a chronic cough. People with CF can inhale DNase through a nebulizer. The cost of the drug is high, and doctors are still trying to come up with guidelines for its use.

Infections: *Staphylococcus* and *Pseudomonas*

Why do infections persist in people with CF? The CF lung, where thickened mucus tends to block the airways, provides a breeding ground for bacteria. And repeated infection can damage the cilia—tiny hairlike projections on the cells that line the lungs and help sweep away particles, debris, and bacteria. So one infection leads to the next. Development of antibiotics that can control infections, particularly *Staphylococcus*, has greatly boosted life expectancy in people with CF. Doctors monitor infections by taking sputum cultures. They collect phlegm, determine which microbes are present in the lungs, and prescribe the antibiotics that are most effective at killing off those organisms.

Antibiotic treatment strategies differ from clinic to clinic. For *Staphylococcus* infection, for example, some doctors prefer aggressively treating the infection with oral antibiotics when it flares up. Others opt for long-term preventive treatment, prescribing lower doses of oral antibiotics all year long. If infections are to be treated only when they occur, parents need to be aware of the signs of infection and bring their children in for treatment right away. This will prevent any extensive lung damage.

In some cases, long-term treatment of an infection with antibiotics will cause the development of bacteria that are no longer killed by the drug. These resistant microbes develop an ability to keep the antibiotics outside their membranes or to chew up and spit out any antibiotic molecules that get in before they can harm the bacteria. Drug-resistant bacteria can also disguise themselves, changing the features on their membranes that an antibiotic would normally recognize so that they're no longer targets. Once a bacterium has figured out how to avoid an antibiotic, it passes this information to its offspring and sometimes to its neighbors. Antibiotic resistance is common for infections of the *Pseudomonas* strains *P. aeruginosa* and *P. cepacia*. Doctors need to administer antibiotics judiciously, so that patients with CF do not develop strains of *Pseudomonas* that are resistant to all common antibiotics.

People with CF usually support infections of *Pseudomonas* their whole lives. Once a person is infected with *Pseudomonas*—particularly *P. cepacia* (also known as *Burkholderia cepacia*)—the bacteria will colonize the respiratory tract and never leave. This bacterium causes serious effects in some and none in others. For all bacteria, the earlier an infection is detected, the easier it is to eliminate with antibiotics.

People with CF generally catch *Pseudomonas aeruginosa* from the environment rather than from another infected person. The bacterium is found everywhere, including in water and soil. Because it is so ubiquitous, *P. aeruginosa* is almost impossible to avoid. Most children with CF are infected by *P. aeruginosa* by the age of 10. On the other hand, people with CF can catch *P. cepacia* from another infected person, so CF clinics often avoid treating patients with *P. cepacia* on the same days when noninfected people are there. Other precautions include isolating infected patients in one area of the intensive care unit or at the clinic and having anyone who is administering medications or conducting ventilator therapy pay meticulous attention to hand washing and sterile techniques.

Controlling *P. cepacia* often requires long-term treatment; some reports suggest that this hardy microbe can survive for years in a bottle of salt water and dilute disinfectant. Some physicians prescribe intermittent treatment with intravenous antibiotics or inhaled antibiotics used over a long period of time. Often doctors prescribe a combined therapy of two antibiotics, because bacteria are less likely to become resistant to both drugs at once. For the double-drug treatment, physicians usually prescribe an *aminoglycoside* antibiotic along with a *penicillin*-like antibiotic. A number of doctors are prescribing an antibiotic called *ciprofloxacin*, particularly for treating *Pseudomonas* infections, but resistance to this drug is becoming more widespread, and it may cause joint pain in some children.

Physiotherapy also helps to control infections by clearing the mucus from the lungs. Clean lungs present a less hospitable home for bacteria, which thrive in the debris and mucus often present in the airways of people with CF.

In general, preventing infections is usually the best course of action. Although people with CF have immune systems that function normally, clearing infections from their lungs is difficult. Parents should make sure that their children with CF receive vaccines to protect them from the most common childhood respiratory infections, such as measles and pertussis (whooping cough). People with CF should also get annual flu shots. While children with CF should avoid unnecessary contact with people who have colds or flu or other contagious illnesses, they should not stay away from school or other activities because they are afraid to catch something. Preventing exposure to germs is virtually impossible, and children need to interact with their peers and the surrounding world to remain physically and emotionally healthy.

DIET AND NUTRITION

Like all children, kids with CF need to follow diets that provide them with adequate nutrition to maintain healthy growth and development. Good nutrition is essential for the promotion of muscle strength and endurance. In addition, children with CF need to consume enough calories so that their lungs can grow and heal properly and their immune systems can fight bacterial infections. A further complication is that most people with CF have pancreatic insufficiency, which thwarts the body's efficient use of nutrients. Because mucous plugs block the digestive enzymes produced by the pancreas from reaching the intestine, a proportion of the calories consumed by children with CF are not absorbed properly. And because children with CF also use extra calories for breathing and battling lung infections, they may need to eat more than other children. For the most part, children with CF consume a regular diet supplemented with enzymes to help them digest their food. If a child with CF has trouble gaining weight, a doctor may prescribe nutritional supplements.

Pancreatic enzyme supplements replace the natural enzymes that get trapped in the pancreas by the mucous plugs that block the pancreatic ducts. The supplements come in the form of capsules or granulated powders that are taken with meals or snacks. The enzymes pass through the stomach and into the intestines, where they help break down food so that it can be absorbed by the small intestine. The pills and granules are coated so that they are resistant to stomach acid and pass undigested through to the intestine. In the small intestine, the enzymes are released, mimicking the natural process of digestion.

The amount of enzymes a person with CF needs to take varies with the age of the individual, the size of the meal, the fat content of the food, and how much damage the disease has done to the pancreas. Most take enzymes with all meals and snacks and, ideally, should take them before or during the meal, not after. The enzymes should allow people with CF to grow normally and to produce normal stools. The most popular enzyme supplements include Pancrease, Creon, and Nutrizym, which contain lipase, amylase, and protease for help in digestion of fats, sugars, and proteins. The enzymes should not be taken with milk, because milk destroys the protective coating on the capsules, allowing the enzymes to be destroyed in the acidic environment of the stomach.

At first, doctors believed that fatty foods should be avoided, because children with CF produce very fatty stools. But fats provide a rich source of calories. And the absorption of fats can be regulated by lipase, a fat-digesting enzyme that is present in the pancreatic enzyme supplements. So, generally speaking, people with the disease do not need to restrict the amount of fat they consume.

People with CF who need enzyme supplements may take an average of 20 pills with every meal. Some of the newer enzyme supplements provide larger amounts of lipase so that fewer pills can be taken at mealtimes. Physicians can offer more advice about which pills are appropriate. Children with CF who need to consume extra calories can also drink high-energy milk shakes as a snack.

Adults and children with CF sometimes do not absorb all the vitamins they need from their food. Dietary supplements, especially of the fat-soluble A, D, E, and K, can replace any vitamins missing in the diet. Insufficient vitamin A can cause dry skin and night blindness. Lack of vitamin K causes bruising and bleeding, and a vitamin E deficiency can result in poor balance. People with CF may also take iron supplements to avoid *anemia*, because iron is part of the *hemoglobin* that transports oxygen to the tissues of the body.

Although it might sound strange, children and adults with CF sometimes need salt supplements, especially in warm weather when they sweat a lot during exercise. Most drink electrolyte solutions to replace any salts or minerals lost during excessive sweating.

Occasionally, thick mucus can cause a backup of stool in the intestine—a condition called *meconium ileus equivalent* or *distal intestinal obstruction syndrome.* Usually the obstruction can be relieved by adjusting the diet and enzyme supplements or flushing the colon with an enema that contains enzymes to help break up the mucus obstruction.

Children and adults with CF who find it impossible to gain weight sometimes undergo an operation called a *button gastrostomy*. This surgical procedure involves the insertion of a small tube into the stomach to allow night feeding of a high-calorie mixture of proteins and fats.

TREATING OTHER SYMPTOMS

If mild diabetes occurs, a person with CF can usually manage the condition by moderating the diet and taking small doses of insulin.

Some people with CF also develop nasal polyps—small outgrowths of mucous membranes inside the nose—which can cause breathing problems because they block the nasal passages. Although physicians can remove these surgically, the polyps often grow back. Applying steroid preparations to the area may help to shrink nasal polyps without surgery.

People with CF can also develop mild problems with their liver function. Doctors sometimes prescribe a drug called ursodeoxycholic acid to help bile acids and salts pass through the liver. By reducing the build-up of bile, doctors can usually improve liver function and prevent cirrhosis.

FERTILITY ISSUES

As we have seen, the majority of men with CF are infertile because the absence of the vas deferens prevents sperm from making it into the ejaculate. In the case of a man with CF who wishes to father children, a physician can collect sperm from the testes with a needle and either introduce it into a woman through artificial insemination or combine it with the woman's eggs in a laboratory dish and then implant the resulting embryos in her uterus. Such manipulations are commonly performed as part of in vitro fertilization.

Women with CF are generally fertile, although thickened mucous secretions around the cervix may make it difficult for sperm to swim to the fallopian tubes, where fertilization takes place. Pregnancy, however, can take a physical toll on women with the disease. The added burden of carrying a baby to term may cause lung function to deteriorate and in some cases can cause heart failure. When considering birth control options, women with CF might want to avoid oral contraceptives, which can cause blood clots, and instead use barrier contraceptives, such as condoms or diaphragms and spermicidal jellies. Physicians, gynecologists, and genetic counselors can offer more advice on pregnancy and contraception.

HOSPITALIZATION

Treatment of chronic bacterial infections in people with CF sometimes requires hospitalization. Physicians usually treat people with severe infections with intravenous antibiotics. The duration of the treatments varies, but people with CF typically remain in the hospital for two to three weeks, until their pulmonary function returns to the preinfection baseline level.

LUNG TRANSPLANTS

In 1985, physicians performed the first lung transplant in the United States. Now more than 400 have been performed nationwide. As of 1996, more than 25 centers in the United States had performed 5 or more lung transplant operations. People with CF who have serious respiratory impairment can opt to receive a lung transplant. Their survival rate is greater than 70 percent in the first year after the surgery. Because the operation is still a relatively new one, physicians do not yet know how much a lung transplant can extend the life of a person with CF.

Donor lungs from healthy individuals do not have CF, because their cells produce a functional CFTR channel protein. Thus someone receiving a lung transplant would no longer experience respiratory difficulties due to CF. Of course, the other organs do not benefit from the surgery, so a person with CF who has problems with digestion must still take dietary enzyme supplements. The biggest problem following transplant is rejection of the donor organ. Someone who receives a transplant must from then on take *immunosuppressant medications* to prevent organ rejection and steroids to fight tissue imflammation.

When lung function deteriorates and traditional physiotherapy and antibiotic treatments no longer improve or maintain respiration, people with CF can get on a waiting list for a lung transplant. Those with the disease usually consider having a transplant when their lung capacity drops to 25 or 30 percent of normal values and their blood carries too little oxygen and too much carbon dioxide; at this point, they are often on oxygen almost full-time.

Lung transplants are not appropriate for every person with late-stage CF. Physicians might exclude a person with CF from receiving a transplant if they think that he or she would be unable to comply with the complicated postoperative recovery program or if there are serious problems in other organs that might compromise the person's ability to survive the operation and the long-term recovery process. Infection with a strain of *P. cepacia* that is resistant to most of the commonly used antibiotics (called pan-resistant *P. cepacia*) may also disqualify a person. Because bacteria can colonize the upper respiratory tract, including the nose and throat, an infection may persist even after surgeons have removed the diseased lungs. After the transplant, the bacteria can then infiltrate the new lungs. Because transplant patients must take medications to suppress their immune systems to avoid rejecting the new organs, any bacteria present stand a better chance of establishing an infection, particularly if they cannot be eliminated by treatment with antibiotics. The policies regarding lung transplants for people infected with pan-resistant *P. cepacia* differ at various transplant centers.

Once a person with CF gets on a waiting list for a lung transplant, he or she should prepare for the operation both physically and mentally. Physicians recommend that the person try to maintain good physical fitness before the surgery. This might be difficult for those who have serious respiratory problems. What is perhaps more important than physical stamina, say people with CF who have successfully undergone transplant surgery, is the need for a "positive attitude toward life." The patients who do the best after the operation are usually highly motivated and have a strong social-support system of family and friends.

Currently, the supply of donor organs cannot meet the demand of those needing transplants; people with other chronic lung ailments are also on the waiting list. The average time between being accepted as a candidate on a waiting list and receiving a lung transplant is more than 18 months at most centers. As more potential donors become aware of the transplant programs, the waiting time should decrease. In future, improvements in *xenotransplantation*—the use of organs from animals such as pigs or baboons—may help alleviate the shortage of human donor organs for transplantation (although use of animal organs in humans remains fairly controversial).

People on a waiting list for a transplant usually carry special pagers that alert them when an organ becomes available. Every person on a transplant waiting list is registered with the United Network for Organ Sharing, which tracks all transplants, donors, and recipients. Once an organ becomes available, time is critical; people on a waiting list usually do what they can to prearrange transportation to the transplant center, as well as making lists of people to call and preparing what they will take to the hospital.

Choosing a transplant center can be confusing. Among the considerations are which center is closest to home, which has the shortest waiting list, and which has the best survival statistics. Even the numbers are not necessarily straightforward. Some centers may prescreen their patients and accept only those with the best chances of long-term survival. People with CF who have had lung transplants recommend talking to others who are on waiting lists or who have had transplants as a way of finding out why one transplant center was chosen and others rejected.

Many people with CF who have received a lung transplant say that the risk and trauma of surgery is worthwhile. After pulmonary rehabilitation, which can include walking on a treadmill and riding a stationary bicycle, people who have received lung transplants find that they can do things they were unable to do before the operation. Within weeks or months of the surgery, people who had barely had the strength to brush their teeth find that they can live life, return to work and school, and enjoy their family and friends. "No more oxygen, face masks, or CPT. I'm biking, walking, swimming, rollerblading—anything you can think of!" wrote one person, describing the transplant experience to an Internet newsgroup for people with CF. "I never realized how great life can be!"

MANAGED CARE ISSUES

According to the Cystic Fibrosis Foundation (CFF), in 1995 the estimated total cost for treating people with CF in the United States topped $900 million. That figure represents an average yearly cost of nearly $40,000 per person with CF.

As more Americans find themselves relying on managed care programs—either health maintenance organizations (HMOs) or preferred provider organizations (PPOs)—paying for health care is becoming a major issue for everyone, not just people with CF. And as managed care providers continue to try to contain costs by tightening their reimbursement policies, people with CF need to be aware of their benefit packages and to learn how to persuade their insurers, when necessary, to pay for the appropriate specialists, treatments, and medications.

You should ask several questions about your health care plan. Can you see your CF center physician if he or she does not belong to your health care network? If so, will your insurer ask you to pay for the visit out-of-pocket? Or will you be responsible for making a higher copayment as a result? (You might be able to get around paying extra for seeing an out-of-network specialist by having your physician join your managed care network.) Does your policy have a lifetime cap on medical care or prescription drugs? Remember, if you disagree with your health care provider about reimbursements, you can ask someone who works in your employer's human resources department to intercede on your behalf. You can also appeal the insurance company's policies directly or file a complaint with your state insurance department.

People with CF should consider supplemental insurance plans that may help to pay for any products or services denied by a managed care organization. State health departments can provide information about Medicaid (for individuals or families with low income) and other programs offered for Children with Special Health Needs (for children under 21 years of age). The Social Security Administration also sponsors some programs that might be of assistance for people with CF. Social security benefits accrue when a person has worked and contributed to the program, and Supplemental Security Income may be available for people who have never held a job. For more information on these programs, contact the Social Security Administration at 1-800-772-1213. Most states sponsor some sort of financial assistance for expenses related to health care. The type of service available usually depends on the family income.

Some pharmaceutical companies provide free medications to those individuals who would otherwise not have access to the drugs. Genentech, Inc., which manufactures the DNase called Pulmozyme, offers three different assistance programs for people with CF. For information about the Pulmozyme program, call 1-800-297-5557. In general, the Pharmaceutical Research and Manufacturers of America can provide a list of pharmacies that offer programs for people with CF. Call 1-800-PMA-INFO for details.

Finally, keep in mind that medical expenses may be tax deductible if they exceed a specified percentage of the family's income and are itemized on the federal tax return. The costs of food supplements may also be deductible. For more information, contact the IRS or a tax advisor.

People with CF should remember that they are their own best advocates when it comes to getting the most from their health care plans. The Cystic Fibrosis Foundation (CFF) can also provide additional suggestions about how to take a more active role in securing and financing the best treatments for CF.

SEEING A DOCTOR

CF centers offer access to specialists who deal specifically with respiratory, digestive, reproductive, and other problems encountered by people with CF. They can also offer counseling services and help people cope with the disease. Physicians who specialize in treating people with CF also often conduct CF-related research. At CF centers, nurses, physical and respiratory therapists, nutritionists, and social workers collaborate with physicians and patients as part of the health care team. (See appendix D for CFF-sponsored care centers in every state.)

Doctors at CF centers also work closely with pediatricians and family physicians to determine the best treatments for a child or an adult with CF. People with CF usually maintain contact with a general practitioner or internist who can treat them when they need a few stitches or are due for a routine physical exam. If people with CF develop other diseases, such as heart disease or cancer, they can be treated by specialists who work outside the CF clinic.

People with CF and their families should learn as much as they can about the disease and about treatment options in order to make informed decisions and to deal most effectively with the situation. They should not be intimidated by the disease or by health care workers. Most physicians appreciate the confusion that this diagnosis can cause and are prepared to give a full explanation of what is involved. Acquiring an understanding of the disease can provide a sense of control to those who have CF, as well as to their caregivers.

CYSTIC FIBROSIS SERVICES, INC.

A subsidiary of CFF, CF Services, Inc., aims to "enhance the quality of life for people with CF by driving down the costs of fighting the disease." Their pharmacy service buys the most commonly used drugs directly from the manufacturers and makes them available to people with CF at up to 40 percent below retail prices. The organization also arranges to ship the medications directly to the home, eliminating the need for people with CF to make multiple trips to the pharmacy.

In addition to its drug services, CF Services, Inc., also acts as an advocate for people with CF, persuading insurance companies and managed care organizations to cover CF therapies. To learn more about CF Services, Inc., call 1-800-541-4959 or visit the CFF web page at *www.cff.org.*

6. Coping with CF

As one who lives daily with the reality of a chronic illness, I have found that seemingly "sick" humor may serve as a means of coping with the spectre of death which looms in my own life. To cope with the reality of death, my family and I participate in what we refer to as Dead Jeff Jokes. These basically take the form of "Jeff, when you die, can I have your . . . ?" where various possessions of mine—my compact-disc player or my car—are inserted at the end of the sentence. Although it sounds downright mean and nasty, this is a legitimate way for our family to cope with the gravity of my illness . . . If you can't laugh at it, what can you do?

Jeffrey Mason, physics major,
Bridgewater State College, Massachusetts

People cope with disease in different ways. Some use humor to deal with difficult situations and to gain some sense of control over the circumstances. Others find comfort in knowledge, seeking to understand the illness by learning everything they can about how it works and what they should expect. Still others derive strength and solace from their spiritual or religious beliefs.

Although improved treatments are prolonging the lives of people with CF, the disease is still chronic and fatal. People with CF and their families learn—from specialists, support groups, and by trial and error—how to live their lives to the fullest and how to prepare for the inevitable. This chapter examines the emotional and psychological impact that CF can have on affected individuals and their friends and families.

DEALING WITH THE DIAGNOSIS

Because CF is usually diagnosed in infancy or early childhood, it is the parents who bear the brunt of the emotional impact. Before a child is diagnosed as having CF, parents may feel anxious and frustrated: their child is suffering and they do not know what is wrong or what they can do to make things better. The actual diagnosis often engenders immediate, if temporary, feelings of relief; at least the parents know what the problem is. And identifying the illness means that doctors can begin medical treatment.

After the initial relief, however, parents are likely to experience a flood of strong and conflicting emotions: concern for the child's well-being, worry about the future, guilt over "giving" a child a serious genetic disease or failing to obtain a diagnosis sooner, resentment about the time and attention the child requires, anger with themselves, their doctors, or their fate, and fear of the unknown—how sick will the child be, how long will the child live, and how will the family cope?

All these emotions are perfectly normal. Many parents find that talking openly about their feelings and fears with family, friends, or other parents helps them to recognize and work through their problems. Health care providers and professionals at the CF clinic can help parents to accept and deal with the diagnosis and the emotions that it evokes. Although it takes time to adjust to a diagnosis of CF, parents need to work through their feelings so that they can provide the child with emotional support.

EMOTIONAL IMPACT OF CF

Coping with a chronic illness on a daily basis can take an emotional toll on the whole family. Parents find that physiotherapy, treatments, and doctors' visits can eat up a great deal of time—time that might otherwise be spent catching up on chores, relaxing, or having fun. Dealing with the disease can cause marital conflicts, limit social interactions, detract from activities with other children in the family, and impose financial burdens.

Because everyone copes with crises differently, parents of a child with CF may find themselves at odds over how to deal with the disease. Each may blame the other for the child's condition or for not seeking medical attention sooner. One or both parents might deny the diagnosis, taking the child from one specialist to another seeking second opinions or alternative explanations. Occasionally a parent, or the person with CF, chooses to believe that the disease might just miraculously disappear, so they dismiss treatment. Some people may experience major depression. Over time, most people coping with CF will find that their moods fluctuate between optimism and despair—at some times they feel in control and at others they feel that they cannot possibly deal with it another day.

Most people find that discussing their feelings and problems with family or close friends helps them keep things in perspective. Interactions with other parents or people with CF—through support groups, CF newsletters, online Internet forums, or the Cystic Fibrosis Foundation—can provide comfort, strength, and perspective. Others may find professional counseling helpful. Learning to recognize and grapple with all the emotions that are associated with such a disease can be difficult. But maintaining a positive attitude certainly helps children with CF accept and cope with their condition and may actually contribute to their good health.

Parents of children with CF or other chronic illnesses may sometimes feel lost, alone, scared, and different from other parents. At the same time, many feel that the disease has helped them focus on the important things in life. "I used to wonder how anyone with a child with a terminal illness could possibly live with that knowledge," wrote one parent to an online CF bulletin board. "After our child was diagnosed, a light came on: We realized that life is a terminal illness and that the only time we really have is now. We just live from day to day, expecting good things."

HOW TO TALK TO A CHILD ABOUT CF

Although it might be difficult, parents should try to remain positive. For example, children can be told that their diagnosis is a good thing: now that the doctor has figured out what has been making them feel bad, they can take some medicine and get some treatments that will make them feel better. Children should be exposed to other people with CF so they can see that they are not alone.

All children ask lots of questions; those with CF are no exception. Parents need to be prepared to answer their children's questions—why they have to take so many pills with their food, why they need physiotherapy, and what they can expect to happen next. Children are often looking for answers that will allay their fears. Parents should try to be honest about CF but avoid leaving their children imagining the worst. Again, pediatricians and counselors can offer advice on how to talk to children about the disease.

CHILDHOOD WITH CF

Childhood can be a complicated time, and having a chronic disease adds to the everyday problems of just being a kid. Parents should try to treat a child with CF as normally as possible; they should avoid being overly protective and should encourage the child to become self-reliant as he or she gets older.

Children with CF may sometimes resist physiotherapy treatments because they intrude on playtime. Therapy need not be a chore, and many parents work toward making treatments a fun part of the family's daily routine. At school, children with CF might find themselves picked on because they are small or because they cough a lot. Some are embarrassed about having to take enzyme tablets with their lunch. Parents should be aware of these potential problems and must keep the lines of communication open, so that children can discuss their feelings or ask for advice.

Parents of children with CF also need to pay special attention to their healthy children. These siblings may sometimes feel neglected and resentful because they get less attention from their parents; one way to keep them from feeling left out is to let them take part in physiotherapy. Siblings may also experience guilt over their feelings or because they are healthy. Many healthy siblings worry about what will happen to them and to their brother or sister with CF. Parents should encourage their children to talk about these feelings and to express their resentment, anger, and fears.

Today, thanks to improved nutrition programs and home treatment protocols, children with CF spend less time out of school and in the hospital than they used to. This makes it easier for kids with CF to be kids.

SURVIVING ADOLESCENCE WITH CF

Teens with CF, like other adolescents, must cope with complex physical, sexual, emotional, and hormonal changes. At a time when youngsters normally strive for independence, autonomy, and privacy, teens with CF also have to come to terms with their dependence on a therapy that may seem strange to their peers. The conflict sometimes causes adolescents to become rebellious and reject their treatments. As adolescents with CF become more conscious of their bodies, they may also find physiotherapy more embarrassing.

Adolescents are painfully concerned with what their peers— particularly those of the opposite sex—think of them. And teens with CF may be pale, underweight, and slow to develop because of their respiratory and digestive difficulties. Adolescence is also a time when many people with CF start to think about the future—their career plans and developing relationships—and when they begin to be concerned about long-term survival.

HOSPITALIZATION

Acute flare-ups of lung infections may occasionally require children with CF to spend a few days or weeks in a hospital. For young children, separation from their parents is the most anxiety-provoking part of the hospital experience. Parents can ask to be allowed to stay in the room with their child. Visits from family or friends can also help the time pass quickly. Toys and any special stuffed animals or books from home can make the hospital experience more entertaining and less frightening. Adolescents with CF sometimes feel uncomfortable staying in a pediatric ward. Some hospitals may offer alternative accommodations, perhaps arranging for teens to share a room.

GROWING OLD WITH CF

Adults with CF come to terms with their disease in different ways. Some accept it as part of their lives, considering the condition to be just another aspect of who they are. Others view CF as a challenge to be overcome. Most try to prevent the disease from dominating their lives. Adults often turn to support groups and networks for camaraderie and an opportunity to discuss their crises and triumphs with other members of the CF community.

Adults with CF hold down full-time or part-time jobs and go to school. Many marry or are involved in long-term relationships; some even start families. As we have seen, pregnancy can be difficult for women with CF, possibly causing deterioration of lung function or even heart failure. And the chances that a baby will die or be born prematurely are greater for women with the disease. In addition, women with CF need to consider the fact that their children might have to grow up without them. For these reasons, many women choose to avoid pregnancy by using contraceptives or undergoing sterilization.

PRENATAL DIAGNOSIS OF CF

People with CF or carriers of CF who opt to have children may want to consider prenatal diagnosis, which involves having a sample of blood or cells taken from the fetus so that its chromosomes can be examined for CF mutations. Doctors can perform amniocentesis to collect cells shed by the fetus, a process that requires removing some of the amniotic fluid that surrounds the developing embryo. They can also draw fetal blood from the umbilical cord or remove a small piece of the chorionic villi, the outer surface of the membrane that surrounds the fetus. Amniocentesis and fetal blood sampling are usually done when the fetus is 16 to 18 weeks old; chorionic villus sampling can be performed earlier in the pregnancy, when the fetus is 8 to 12 weeks old.

Making a decision about whether to continue or terminate a pregnancy on the basis of a prenatal diagnostic screen is extremely difficult. Although CF can be treated, some parents might not wish to sentence a child to a life with a chronic, fatal disease. Genetic counselors can help couples review their options and live with their decisions.

FACING DEATH

Many books have been written on the subject of dealing with death and dying. People with CF have to come to grips with their own mortality, and parents have to prepare themselves for the death of a child. Although parents might not always express their fears at the moment, many say that with each infection they wonder whether it will be the one that marks the beginning of the end.

According to psychologists, children do not really see death as a permanent and inevitable event until they are about 10 years old. As children with CF get older and come to realize that the disease is ultimately fatal, they may experience depression or anxiety. Some may develop feelings of impending death and may go through a stage of isolation, as if to prepare for separation. Most children respond best to the truth and should be allowed to ask questions about what they can expect to happen.

When the end is near, a person with CF should choose whether to die at home or in the hospital. Doctors can provide medications to keep a person who is near death as comfortable as possible. Intravenous sedatives can help the person relax and remain calm, and morphine can relieve any pain and also help a person with CF feel that he or she can breathe more easily (even though the drug actually suppresses breathing).

Letting go of a loved one is never easy, especially when the loved one is a child. "Her dad spent a lot of time with her in her last two days just talking. She was asleep most of the time," wrote one mother about her daughter's final days. "He spoke to her about the perfect place and what it would be like: not having cystic fibrosis, having a perfect set of lungs, and being able to run with her dog Nissy all day, every day."

Every person who experiences such a loss goes through a period of grief and mourning. Some find comfort in family and friends, others in religion or counseling. Most enjoy remembering how loving a person with CF made their lives richer.

"Sarah was in our lives for 10 3/4 years and taught us a lot," wrote one mother. "We learnt the value of the simple things in life, like being together and loving each other. We learnt to pull together in difficult times and not shut each other out. We learnt that no person is an island and how much we need each other. We learnt how much we love our children and how we must never take them for granted. We are grateful to God for giving us such a wonderful, special child."

7. Future Treatments, Potential Cures

The fact that many groups are now studying gene therapy for CF in humans is remarkable. Remember, the gene was only discovered a few years ago. I think we're definitely moving in the right direction toward finding a cure.

Ronald Crystal, Cornell University Medical Center,

who performed the first human gene therapy experiment

for CF in 1993

Right now, there is no cure for CF. Decades-old therapies are still used to treat the most serious symptoms of the disease. Doctors prescribe thumping on the backs of CF patients to help dislodge the thick mucus that builds up in their lungs and antibiotics to manage the chronic infections that often eventually lead to respiratory failure. Digestive enzyme supplements help people with CF to digest their food.

But scientists are using their understanding of the biology of CF to develop more elegant therapies that would correct the fundamental defect—the loss of activity of the CFTR ion channel in the cell membrane that leads to impaired chloride flow and to the accumulation of thick mucus in the lungs, pancreas, and other organs. If researchers could devise a way to restore the proper movement of chloride ions into and out of the critical cells, they would essentially eradicate the symptoms of CF.

Many groups of scientists are searching for such a treatment. Because the mucus buildup in the lungs of people with CF causes life-threatening infections and respiratory problems, scientists are aiming their molecular therapies at the epithelial cells lining the bronchial airways. *Gene therapy*, if it can be made more effective, would provide the most direct approach for relieving the problems caused by a defective CFTR protein. Such therapy would somehow introduce the normal CFTR gene into the proper lung airway epithelial cells.

Scientists are currently conducting CFTR gene therapy trials in humans, but it will be years before they figure out whether the treatments are safe, efficient, and effective. Until then, other teams of scientists are approaching the problem from a different perspective—trying to design drugs that will correct the chloride channel defect and restore the proper ion balance to the critical cells.

One way scientists may be able to reestablish the flow of chloride ions in epithelial cells is to somehow revive the defective CFTR protein, making it behave more like normal CFTR. Remember, some CFTR mutations direct cells to make a CFTR channel that does not work as effectively as the normal channel. Perhaps scientists can design drugs that will switch these mutant CFTR channels on. Other mutations, including the most common, ΔF508, cause the CFTR protein to get stuck in the cell cytoplasm and become degraded before it reaches the membrane where it can perform its molecular duties. Some scientists are looking for drugs that can help escort this defective CFTR protein to the cell membrane, where it might be able to function well enough to keep the cell healthy. Fortunately, scientists think that cells might be able to function normally with as little as 10 to 20 percent of the normal CFTR activity.

But restoring CFTR activity is not the only path to more effective treatments. Other scientists are trying to design ways to get around the CFTR defect by activating another channel that could perform the same molecular job, allowing chloride ions to pass into or out of the appropriate cells. Still other researchers are trying to learn more about the natural antibiotic that lung epithelial cells produce to eliminate the microbes that enter the airways with every breath. Some experiments suggest that the salt that accumulates in the mucus clogging the lungs of people with CF disables that natural antibiotic, allowing incoming bacteria to thrive. If researchers can figure out how to replace the antibiotic, a molecule called *beta-defensin*, or make it work in the presence of salt, they might be able to help people with CF combat bacterial infections.

How feasible are these experimental approaches? And when might they move from the laboratory to the clinic? Let's examine each and assess the possibilities.

GENE THERAPY

Because CF is caused by defects in a single gene, researchers consider it a prime candidate for treatment by gene therapy. By delivering the normal CFTR gene to the defective cells, scientists could effectively cure CF. In fact, soon after they discovered the CFTR gene, scientists found that they could restore chloride-channel activity to cells from CF patients in a culture dish by adding the normal CFTR gene.

Again, because the most serious CF symptoms involve the lungs, scientists are exploring ways to introduce a single copy of the normal CFTR gene into lung epithelial cells. Remember, just one copy of the normal gene will enable a cell to make enough CFTR protein to keep that cell healthy: carriers do not have CF. But how do scientists deliver genes to the target cells? Genes cannot be taken orally, in a pill, like a regular drug. They have to be inserted directly into the proper cell. Fortunately, doctors have fairly easy access to lung epithelial cells because they are exposed to the outside world. Drugs in aerosol mists can be applied directly to cells that line the airways.

To get the genes into the lung cells, scientists take advantage of the biology of viruses. Although we usually think of viruses as the enemy because they make us sick, their ability to infect human cells makes them particularly useful to scientists trying to develop gene therapy strategies. Like humans and other animals, viruses also carry their genes on chromosomes made of DNA or its relative, ribonucleic acid (RNA). A virus infects a human cell by injecting its genetic material—DNA or RNA, depending on the virus—into the cell like a tiny molecular syringe.

To harness this natural talent of viruses, scientists introduce human genes, such as CFTR, into a virus. If this modified virus then infects a patient, it will deliver the CFTR gene, along with its own genetic material, into the patient's cells. And because scientists working on gene therapy for CF need to get the CFTR gene into lung cells, they use a modified *adenovirus* as a delivery vehicle. As one of the viruses that causes the common cold, the adenovirus is fond of infecting airway cells. It already has the specialized equipment it needs to gain access to lung epithelial cells—like a burglar who has the right tools to crack a bank safe. So scientists insert the CFTR gene into adenovirus and remove the viral genes that normally allow it to take over a cell and reproduce itself.

Right now, scientists administer the doctored virus to patients in experimental trials in nose drops or by drizzling it down the back of the throat using a bit of flexible tubing called a *bronchoscope*. In the future, physicians would like to introduce the CFTR-carrying adenovirus in an aerosol mist that gets sprayed into the lungs with an infuser like the ones asthmatics use to inhale the drugs that relax their constricted airways.

The U.S. Congress has granted the National Institutes of Health (NIH) about $40 million to establish the nine CF gene therapy centers listed in appendix D. The Cystic Fibrosis Foundation has provided an additional $10 million for developing gene therapy for CF. In 1993, Ron Crystal, then working at NIH, performed the first gene therapy treatment on a patient with CF. By early 1997, scientists had initiated seven different clinical trials designed to determine whether CFTR gene therapy is safe and effective. Six of the studies involve adenovirus; these are being performed at Cornell University, the University of Iowa, the University of Washington, the University of Pennsylvania, the University of North Carolina, the University of Cincinnati, and the Massachusetts General Hospital. Meanwhile, researchers at the University of Alabama are conducting gene therapy trials using fat capsules called *liposomes* rather than adenovirus to deliver the CFTR gene. And researchers at the Johns Hopkins University School of Medicine recently initiated a clinical trial using the related *adeno-associated virus* to deliver CFTR to the lung cells of people with CF. By June 1997, nearly 150 CF patients in the United States had received gene therapy treatment.

None of these trials has gone on long enough to tell scientists whether their CF gene therapy strategies will be successful. Clinical trials usually run for two to four years and go through three phases. Then the Food and Drug Administration (FDA) has to approve the protocol for the marketplace, which usually takes another couple of years. All the CF gene therapy trials are currently in Phase I of the three phases of this process, in which scientists test the safety and efficiency of their strategy.

Problems with gene therapy

Though the method sounds fairly straightforward, gene therapy protocols have run into some problems in the clinic. Engineered viruses can transfer their genetic cargo efficiently in cell cultures, but researchers have found that accomplishing the same feat in a human being is a bit more difficult. First, the viruses have to get past the mucus in the lungs, which forms a physical barrier that blocks access to the cells lining the airways. Next, the virus has to find the right epithelial cells, the ones that normally use CFTR to expel chloride ions. These are not necessarily lying in wait at the surface of the lung, but line the mucous glands in the airways (fig 4.2).

A number of researchers, including Crystal and his collaborators at GenVec, Inc., in Rockville, Maryland, are working on bolstering the ability of adenovirus to penetrate lung epithelial cells. Any manipulations that improve the accuracy and efficiency of the viral delivery system will dramatically improve the chances that the CFTR gene will get into the correct cells.

The other problem with using viruses to deliver the CFTR gene is that the outer structure of viruses, which surrounds the viral DNA or RNA like a molecular container, is made of proteins. Foreign proteins can evoke an immune response that will clear the invading virus from the body and may make the lungs even more inflamed than they would be in a person with untreated CF. Even if the virus itself escapes immediate detection, the body's immune system may target the epithelial cells infected with the virus for destruction, eliminating the very cells that have received the CFTR gene. To get around this problem, scientists, including James Wilson and his colleagues at the University of Pennsylvania in Philadelphia, are designing more stealthy viruses—ones that will be able to slip past the immune system and deliver the genes without getting noticed. This involves paring down the virus as much as possible to get rid of the viral proteins that might catch the attention of the immune system.

Another way to prevent the adenovirus carrying CFTR from being destroyed would be to administer it along with a drug that suppresses a patient's normal immune response to the virus. This immunosuppressant drug should prevent the body from generating antibodies to the adenovirus—a reaction that often makes readministration of the gene in the same type of virus impossible. Such drugs already exist and are used to prevent the rejection of transplanted organs.

Some scientists have elected to avoid the problems involved in using viruses entirely. Instead, these researchers encase the CFTR gene in little bubbles of fat, or lipid. These liposomes transport the CFTR gene to the surface of a cell and then, because cell membranes are also made mostly of lipids, the liposomes fuse with the cell like two soap bubbles joining to make a larger bubble. When that happens, the liposome spills its contents—the CFTR gene—into the cell. This method is likely to be less efficient than using virus, but may not produce the side effects associated with the immune response.

Both these methods of delivering genes share other problems. Even if the CFTR gene gets into the proper cell in the airway, as part of the normal process of cell turnover that keeps tissues healthy, these cells will die and be replaced by cells that have not received a copy of the normal CFTR genes. So gene therapy might have to be repeated every few months in order to maintain a stockpile of cells that have the normal CFTR gene.

DRUG THERAPIES

Although gene therapy holds great promise for the future, pharmacological therapies that relieve CF symptoms may prove more practical in the short term. As we have seen, many patients with CF currently use an aerosolized drug called DNase, approved by the FDA in 1994, to loosen the thick mucus in their lungs. The enzyme degrades the sticky strands of DNA that spill out of cells killed by the immune response to chronic airway infections. Drugs such as DNase are much easier to administer than gene therapy and have fewer problems finding their way to the proper cells.

Most potential drug therapies currently under investigation aim to activate a chloride channel—either CFTR or a related channel—in the epithelial cells of people with CF.

Helping mutant CFTR to the cell membrane

Of the 700 different mutations in the CFTR gene that lead to CF, one class of mutations, present in 5 percent of people with CF, causes the production of truncated, nonfunctional CFTR proteins that never make it to the cell membrane. In these premature-stop mutants, a molecular stop signal appears in the middle of the CFTR gene. If scientists could encourage the cellular machinery that adds amino acids to the growing protein to read through that stop signal, insert another amino acid, and continue making the protein, the cell should be able to produce a full-length CFTR channel that gets inserted into the cell membrane.

In fact, certain antibiotics, called aminoglycosides, can fool the protein-making machinery into doing just that. It's a trick that David Bedwell of the University of Alabama in Birmingham and his colleagues think might someday prove useful in treating CF. When the researchers exposed cells carrying the mutant CFTR gene to an aminoglycoside antibiotic called G-418, the cells produced roughly 25 to 35 percent as much full-length CFTR protein as did the cells that expressed the normal CFTR protein. Thus G-418 appeared to override the stop signal with some degree of efficiency. And the slightly imperfect CFTR protein produced by these cells actually works: it can expel chloride ions from the cell. Bedwell finds the results encouraging, because CF researchers generally believe that restoring as little as 10 percent of normal CFTR activity might alleviate the symptoms of the disease. As of 1997, Bedwell and his colleagues were currently recruiting patients to test the safety of aminoglycosides in treating CF in Phase I trials that were just getting under way.

Other researchers are trying to find ways to coax mutant ΔF508 CFTR proteins to the cell membrane. This mutation, the most common in people with CF, prevents the CFTR protein from folding into its proper shape, leaving it stranded in the cell cytoplasm where it gets destroyed by the cell's molecular cleanup machinery. Scientists at the Johns Hopkins University School of Medicine in Baltimore have shown that a drug called phenylbutyrate can help ΔF508 CFTR assume its proper shape and insert into the membrane in CF cells in a culture dish in the laboratory. In 1997, the researchers were also recruiting volunteers who have two copies of the ΔF508 mutation to participate in a Phase I trial to test this drug.

Normal CFTR channel proteins can be switched on by a chemical modification called *phosphorylation*—the addition of a phosphate molecule to a protein. Certain enzymes in the cell perform this phosphorylation, which turns the CFTR protein on. And other enzymes, called *phosphatases*, undo the phosphorylation, effectively shutting CFTR channels down. Scientists led by John Hanrahan of McGill University in Montreal, Canada, have figured out a way to take advantage of this natural cellular regulatory system to help keep mutant CFTR proteins turned on. For a certain class of CFTR mutations, the mutant proteins make it to the cell membrane but are not as active as normal CFTR. The Canadian researchers found that they could stimulate the activity of mutant CFTR channels by chemically blocking the phosphatase enzymes that would normally shut them off.

Activating alternative chloride channels

The CFTR protein isn't the only fish in the chloride-channel sea. When it comes to normalizing the flow of chloride in the epithelial cells of CF patients, researchers led by Richard Boucher at the University of North Carolina in Chapel Hill have found that any chloride-ion channel worth its salt might do the job. In 1996, Boucher and his colleagues demonstrated that a simple drug therapy could activate an alternative chloride-ion channel in the lungs of CF patients, which would allow them to eliminate infectious microbes and other particles from their airways despite the absence of CFTR.

The drug, called *uridine triphosphate* or *UTP*, may help to restore the proper chloride-ion balance to the airways by directly stimulating this alternative, calcium-activated chloride-ion channel or by activating the tiny, hairlike cilia on lung epithelial cells that help to sweep bacteria and other particles away. In either case, Boucher says that proof of UTP's therapeutic benefits will have to await more lengthy clinical trials. Again, in

1997 the researchers were seeking volunteers for Phase I clinical trials to test UTP and another drug called amiloride for their ability to relieve the symptoms of CF.

Turning to a natural antibiotic

In 1996, a group of researchers led by Jeffrey Smith and Michael Welsh at the University of Iowa College of Medicine in Iowa City discovered that the salty mucus present in the lungs of people with CF directly impairs their ability to fight off bacterial infections by inactivating a natural antibiotic produced by lung epithelial cells. Without the help of this antibiotic molecule, epithelial cells from the lungs of CF patients cannot clear the thousands of microbes that are swept into the airways with each and every breath (fig. 7.1).

In 1997, researchers led by Michael Zasloff of Magainin Pharmaceuticals in Maryland showed that the natural antibiotic crippled by high salt is a peptide called beta-defensin—a small protein similar to antibiotics produced by the skin of frogs. Now that researchers have identified the protective molecule, they can try to modify it so that it can function in the high-salt conditions present in the lungs of people with CF. If they succeed, the researchers might be able to aerosolize the antibiotic and use it as a treatment for eliminating the infections that damage the lungs of people with CF. The therapy would enable the cells lining the lungs to destroy invading microbes, such as *Pseudomonas aeruginosa* and *Staphylcoccus aureus*, even in the absence of CFTR.

CONCLUSIONS

Scientists and physicians remain hopeful that one or more of the therapies described here will someday offer a cure for people with CF. Researchers are currently testing these therapies in ongoing clinical trials and in many cases are still recruiting subjects. Although each trial has specific requirements, in

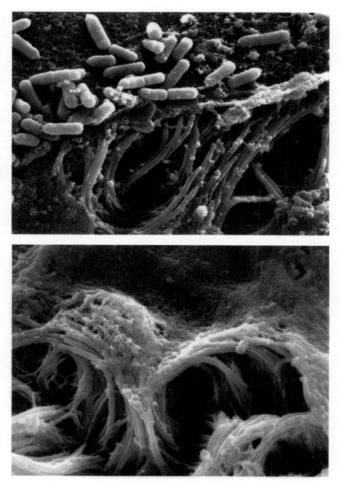

FIG. 7.1. Natural antibiotics may help people with CF fight infections. In people with CF, the high concentration of salt in the mucus that coats the epithelial cells lining the lungs may inactivate a natural antibiotic that helps kill inhaled microbes. Pictures taken by a scanning-electron microscope show that bacteria such as *Pseudomonas aeruginosa* thrive in the high-salt environment produced by epithelial cells from a CF patient (top). When researchers wash away the salt, the natural antibiotic produced by the epithelial cells destroys the bacteria (bottom). (Reproduced with permission from Jeffrey Smith, University of Iowa.)

general, volunteers must be 14 to 18 years of age or older to participate. Some studies request that patients be in good health or have a certain level of lung function. To find out more about taking part in a CF clinical trial—and becoming part of the search for the cure—contact the Cystic Fibrosis Foundation in Bethesda, Maryland (see appendix C).

Appendices

Knowledge is power, and people with CF and others interested in the disease have access to an increasing number of excellent sources of information. National and international CF organizations can provide literature on the biology of CF and its diagnosis and treatment, as well as up-to-date information on the latest research. For people with access to the Internet, these foundations, along with a number of nonprofit organizations, offer detailed information and references online. In addition, newsletters provide updated information either electronically or through the mail. Following are some of the most informative resources and a list of the CF centers in the United States.

APPENDIX A: THE INTERNET

We live in the Information Age, and anyone with a computer modem can easily access data electronically, with the press of a button or the click of a mouse. People interested in learning more about CF can access any number of fine sources and become informed about everything from the history of CF to the sequences of the CFTR gene and protein to the mutations that cause CF. Many electronic sites are maintained by scientists who use the Internet (also known as the World Wide Web) as a way to make their data available to others and to access information collected on CF from around the world. Other sites offer a place for people with CF, and their families and friends, to chat about their questions or concerns.

Because anyone with a modem can post information electronically, without regard to accuracy, always check any information obtained from an Internet site with a reliable source—a doctor, a published book or article about CF, or a Web site that is maintained by a certified CF organization or hospital.

Clearinghouse sites

The CF Web Home Page is a good place to start when searching for any information on CF. Located at *http://www.ai.mit.edu/people/mernst/cf*, the CF Web offers an excellent index of CF-related Internet sites and a fairly comprehensive listing of support services available for people in the CF community. Established by Rob Calhoun, a graduate student at the Massachusetts Institute of Technology in Cambridge, the CF Web also provides an extensive archive of information contributed by people with CF and their families and friends.

Scientific sites

A number of sites offer the full sequence of the CFTR gene, detailed information about the structure and function of the CFTR channel protein, and extensive references on the current research in CF biology and genetics. Two such sites include the Online Mendelian Inheritance in Man (OMIM) database and the Cystic Fibrosis Mutation database.

The National Center for Biotechnology Information developed the OMIM database to catalogue all human genes and genetic disorders. This database, authored and edited by Victor McKusick and his colleagues at Johns Hopkins University and elsewhere, can be found at *http://www3.ncbl.nlm.nih.gov/omim/*. The site offers a comprehensive source of information, including a thorough synopsis of the clinical symptoms and pathologies related to CF, a full history of the medical and scientific breakthroughs that have led to a fuller understanding of the disease, and descriptions of many of the mutations that cause CF.

The Cystic Fibrosis Mutation Database, located at *http://www.genet.sickkids.on.ca/cftr,* was compiled by Lap-Chee Tsui of the Hospital for Sick Children in Toronto from information collected by the Cystic Fibrosis Genetic Analysis Consortium. The site includes figures that reveal the locations and prevalence of the most common CFTR mutations and the full sequence of the CFTR gene. It also provides links to CF newsletters and to other useful CF resources.

APPENDIX B: SUPPORT GROUPS, NEWSLETTERS, AND MAILING LISTS

The most comprehensive Internet support group is the Cystic-L Community page, which can be found at *http://www.ai.mit.edu/people/mernst/cf/cystic-l.* Established in 1994 as an electronic forum for discussion of issues that concern people affected by CF, the site has grown into a small and welcoming virtual community where people ask for advice, pass along knowledge, and share news. People with CF and their families and friends can turn to Cystic-L for some scientific and medical information as well as for stimulating discussions about living with the disease. Cystic-L member Ron Trueworthy has compiled a comprehensive summary of frequently asked questions (CF-FAQ) which can be downloaded onto one's computer.

In addition to the Cystic-L group, many nonprofit organizations offer access to information about CF. A few are listed below, along with the relevant contact information.

The Cystic Fibrosis Alliance is an all-volunteer, nonprofit organization of people with CF, their families, friends, and health care providers. For more information, write to PO Box 4213, Ft. Lauderdale, FL 33338 or call (305) 463-4440.

CF Network, Inc., a nonprofit organization for adults with CF in the United States, publishes a quarterly newsletter called *Network.* For subscription information, send an e-mail note to editor Larry Culp at *LDCulp@voicenet.com* or write to CF Network, Inc., PO Box 3459 Littleton, CO.

The International Association of Cystic Fibrosis Adults, a nonprofit organization run by Adults with Cystic Fibrosis, connects people with CF around the world with one another and with members of the medical community. The association also publishes a quarterly newsletter. For information, contact Barbara Palys, 82 Ayer Road, Harvard, Boston, Massachusetts 01451 or visit the organization's Internet site at *http://ourword.compuserve.com/homepages/FAntognini/ iacfa.htm.*

Michael Jorda runs the mailing list for the International Mucoviscidosis Association. To subscribe, send the message "Subscribe CYSTIC FIBROSIS" to *listserv@frmopII.cnusc.fr.*

The United States Adult Cystic Fibrosis Foundation publishes a newsletter called *CF Roundtable.*

APPENDIX C: CF ORGANIZATIONS

Many national and international organizations can provide up-to-date information about the biology, genetics, and treatment of CF. Most contribute financially to the search for a cure for CF and to the improvement of current treatments and education of the public about the disease. For more information, contact any of the major CF organizations or any one of the local CF care centers, listed alphabetically by state.

Cystic Fibrosis Foundation (CFF)
6931 Arlington Road
Bethesda, Maryland 20814
800-FIGHT-CF
(301) 951-4422
http://www.cff.org

Canadian Cystic Fibrosis Foundation
2221 Yonge Street
Suite 601
Toronto, Ontario
Canada M4S 2B4
(416) 485-9149
http://www.ccfa.ca/~cfwww/toc.html

Cystic Fibrosis Trust
Alexandra House
5 Blyth Road
Bromley, Kent
BR1 3RS
United Kingdom
011-44-181-464-7211
http://www.child-health.dundee.
ac.uk/cf-server/cftrust/index.htm

International Cystic Fibrosis
(Mucoviscidosis) Association
Fliederweg 45
CH-3138
Uetendorf, Switzerland
011-41-31-324-1170
http://tron.is.s.u-tokyo.ac.jp/WHO/
programmes/ina/ngo/ngo-57.htm

APPENDIX D: CFF RESEARCH AND TREATMENT CENTERS

In the United States, CFF coordinates more than 120 treatment centers and provides funding to 9 centers that conduct CF research and gene therapy trials.

CF research centers

University of Alabama at Birmingham
Center Director: Eric Sorscher, M.D.
796 BHSB 1918 University Boulevard
UAB Station
Birmingham, AL 35294-0005

University of California, San
 Francisco*
Center Director: Alan Verkman,
 M.D., Ph.D.
Box 0532
San Francisco, CA 94143-0532
Gene therapy: Center director: Y.W.
 Kan, M.D., F.R.S.
U 426
San Francisco, CA 94143-0724

University of Iowa*
Center Director: Michael Welsh,
 M.D.
Division of Pulmonary Diseases
Howard Hughes Medical Institute
500 ERMB
Iowa City, IA 52242

Johns Hopkins University School of
 Medicine*
Center Director: William Guggino,
 Ph.D.
725 North Wolfe Street
Wood Basic Science Building,
 Room 212
Baltimore, MD 21205-2185

University of North Carolina at
 Chapel Hill*
Center Director: Richard Boucher,
 M.D.
724 Burnett-Womack Building
 CB #7020
Chapel Hill, NC 27599-7020
Gene therapy: 7011 Thurston-Bowles
 Building, CB #7248

Children's Hospital Medical Center*
Center Director: Jeffrey Whitsett,
 M.D.
Children's Hospital Research
 Foundation
3333 Burnet Avenue
Cincinnati, OH 45229-3039

Case Western Reserve University
Center Director: Pamela Davis, M.D.,
 Ph.D.
2101 Adelbert Road
Cleveland, OH 44106

University of Pennsylvania Medical
 Center*
Center Director: James Wilson, M.D.,
 Ph.D.
The Wistar Institute, Room 204
36th and Spruce Streets
Philadelphia, PA 19104-4268

University of Washington*
Center Director: Bonnie Ramsey,
M.D.
Children's Hospital and Medical
Center
4800 Sand Point Way N.E.
PO Box C5371
Seattle, WA 98105

* Research centers marked with an
asterisk are also CFF/NIH gene
therapy centers. Any differences in
contact information are noted.

In addition, the following centers are
involved in gene therapy trials:

Cornell Medical Center
Center Director: Ronald Crystal,
M.D.
520 East 70th Street, Suite 505
New York, NY 10021

Institute for Molecular Genetics
Center Director: Arthur Beaudet,
M.D.
Baylor College of Medicine
One Baylor Plaza, T-619
Houston, TX 77030

CF treatment centers in the United States and Puerto Rico

ALABAMA
Birmingham
UAB Cystic Fibrosis Center
The Children's Hospital
University of Alabama at Birmingham
Appts: (205) 939-9583
Center Director: Raymond Lyrene,
M.D.

Mobile
USA Children's Medical Center
Appts: (334) 343-6848
Center Director: Lawrence J. Sindel,
M.D.

ARIZONA
Phoenix
Cystic Fibrosis Center
Phoenix Children's Hospital
Appts: (602) 239-6925
Center Director: Peggy J. Radford,
M.D.

Tucson
Tucson Cystic Fibrosis Center
St. Luke's Chest Clinic
Arizona Health Sciences Center
Appts: (520) 694-7450
Center Director: Wayne J. Morgan,
M.D.

ARKANSAS
Little Rock
Arkansas Cystic Fibrosis Center
Arkansas Children's Hospital
Appts: (501) 320-1018
Center Director: Robert H. Warren,
M.D.
Adult Program Director: Paula
Anderson, M.D.

CALIFORNIA
Long Beach
Cystic Fibrosis Center
Memorial Miller Children's Hospital
Appts: (310) 933-3290
Center Director: Eliezer Nussbaum,
M.D.

Satellite Center: Ventura County
Medical Center
Appts: (805) 652-6124
Director: Chris Landon, M.D.

Los Angeles
Cystic Fibrosis Comprehensive
Center
Children's Hospital of Los Angeles
Appts: (213) 669-2287 (direct line),
(213) 660-2450 (hospital)
Center Director: C. Michael Bowman,
M.D., Ph.D.

Adult Program: University of
Southern California, Ambulatory
Health Care Center
Appts: (213) 342-5100
Director: Bertrand Shapiro, M.D.

Satellite Center: Kaiser-Permanente
Southern California
Appts: (818) 375-2909 (ask for Linda
Barraza; open to members of the
Kaiser-Permanente Health Plan
only)
Director: Allan S. Lieberthal, M.D.

Outreach: Cedars Sinai Medical
Center
Appts: (310) 855-4433
Co-directors: C. Michael Bowman,
M.D., Ph.D. (children), Andrew
Wachtel, M.D. (adults)

Oakland
Kaiser Permanente Medical Center
Attn: Gail Farmer, R.D.
Department of Pediatrics
Appts: (510) 596-6906 (ask for Gail
Farmer)
Center Director: Gregory F. Shay,
M.D.
(Kaiser has four locations; call Gail
Farmer for information.)

Pediatric Pulmonary Center
Children's Hospital-Oakland
Appts: (510) 428-3305
Center Director: Nancy C. Lewis,
M.D.

Orange
Cystic Fibrosis and Pediatric
Pulmonary Care, Teaching, and
Resource Center
Children's Hospital of Orange County
Appts: (714) 532-8317
Center Director: David Hicks, M.D.

Palo Alto
Stanford Cystic Fibrosis Center
Lucile Packard Children's Hospital at
Stanford
Appts: (415) 497-8841 (scheduling),
(415) 497-8845 (coordinator)
Center Director: Richard Moss, M.D.

Satellite Center: California Pacific
Medical Center
Department of Pediatrics
Director: Karen A. Hardy, M.D.

Sacramento
Cystic Fibrosis and Pediatric
Respiratory Diseases Center
University of California at Davis
School of Medicine
Department of Pediatrics
Appts: (916) 734-3112
Center Director: Ruth McDonald,
M.D.
Adult Program Director: Carroll
Cross, M.D.

San Bernardino
Brian Wesley Ray Cystic Fibrosis
Center
San Bernardino County Medical
Center
Department of Pediatrics
Appts: (909) 387-8155 or (909) 387-7705
Center Director: Gerald R. Greene,
M.D., M.P.H.
Adult Program Director: Mark
Robinson, M.D.

San Diego
San Diego Cystic Fibrosis and
Pediatric Pulmonary Disease
Center
UCSD Medical Center
Appts: (619) 294-6125
Center Director: Michael Light, M.D.

San Francisco
Cystic Fibrosis Center
University of California at San
Francisco
Room M650
Appts: (415) 476-2072
Center Director: Gerd J.A. Cropp,
M.D., Ph.D.
Adult Program Director: Michael S.
Stulbarg, M.D.

Satellite Center: Valley Children's
Hospital, Pediatric Pulmonary
and Respiratory Care
Appts: (209) 243-5550
Director: R. Sudhakar, M.D.

COLORADO
Denver
Denver Children's Hospital
Appts: (303) 837-2522
Center Director: Frank J. Accurso,
M.D.
Adult Program Director: David
Rodman, M.D.

University of Colorado
Appts: (303) 270-7047

Satellite Center: Billings Clinic
Appts: (406) 238-2310
Director: Nicholas Wolter, M.D.

CONNECTICUT
Hartford
Cystic Fibrosis Center
Pediatric Pulmonology Division
Connecticut Children's Medical
Center
Appts: (860) 545-9440
Center Director: Michelle Cloutier,
M.D.

New Haven
Cystic Fibrosis Center
Yale University School of Medicine
Appts: (203) 785-2480
Center Director: Regina Palazzo,
M.D.

DISTRICT OF COLUMBIA
Washington, D.C.
Metropolitan D.C. Cystic Fibrosis
Center for Care, Training and
Research
Children's National Medical Center
Appts: (202) 884-2128
Center Director: Robert J. Fink, M.D

FLORIDA
Gainesville
Cystic Fibrosis and Pediatric
Pulmonary Disease Center
University of Florida
Appts: (352) 392-4458
Center Director: Mary H. Wagner,
M.D.
Adult Program Director: Arundhati
Foster, M.D.

Jacksonville
Nemours Children's Clinic
Appts: (904) 390-3788
Center Director: Ian Nathanson,
M.D.

Orlando
Cystic Fibrosis Center
Orlando Regional Medical Center
Appts: (407) 237-6327
Center Director: Joseph J. Chiaro,
M.D.

St. Petersburg
Cystic Fibrosis Center
All Children's Hospital
Appts: (813) 892-4146
Center Director: Michelle
Howenstine, M.D.

Adult Program: University of South
Florida
Pulmonology Critical Care
Appts: (813) 892-4146
Director: Mark Rolfe, M.D.

Satellite Centers: St. Mary's Hospital, Inc.
Appts: (407) 881-2911
Director: Sue Goldfinger, M.D.
Division of Pulmonology
Miami Children's Hospital
Appts: (305) 662-8380
Director: Carlos Diaz, M.D.
University of South Florida
Department of Pediatrics
Division of Pulmonology
College of Medicine
Appts: (813) 276-5520
Director: Bruce M. Schnapf, D.O.

Outreach Clinics: New Port Richey Specialty Care Clinic
Sarasota Clinic
Tampa Clinic
Appts: (813) 892-4146

GEORGIA
Atlanta
Emory University Cystic Fibrosis Center
Department of Pediatrics
Appts: (404) 727-5728
Center Director: Daniel B. Caplan, M.D.

Augusta
Department of Pediatrics
Section of Pulmonology
Medical College of Georgia
Appts: (706) 721-2635
Center Director: Lou Guill, M.D.
Adult Program Director: John DuPre, M.D.

Satellite Center: Scottish Rite Children's Medical Center
Director: Peter H. Scott, M.D.

Outreach Clinic: Ware County Health Department
Appts: (912) 283-1875

HAWAII: See Tripler Army Medical Center (Fort Sam Houston, Texas)

IDAHO: See University of Utah Medical Center (Nampa and S.E. Idaho)

ILLINOIS
Chicago
Cystic Fibrosis Center
Children's Memorial Hospital
Northwestern University
Appts: (312) 880-4382
Center Director: Susanna A. McColley, M.D.

Wyler Children's Hospital
Department of Pediatrics
University of Chicago Hospitals and Clinics
Appts: (312) 702-6178
Center Director: Lucille A. Lester, M.D.

Rush-Presbyterian-St. Luke's Medical Center
Appts: (312) 942-2889
Center Director: John D. Lloyd-Still, M.D.

Department of Pediatrics
Loyola University Medical Center
Appts: (708) 327-9117
Center Director: Harold Conrad, M.D.

Park Ridge
Cystic Fibrosis Center
Lutheran General Children's Hospital
Victor Yacktman Children's Pavilion
Appts: (847) 318-9330
Center Director: Jerome R. Kraut, M.D.
Adult Program Director: Arvey Stone, M.D.

Peoria
Cystic Fibrosis Center
Saint Francis Medical Center
  Specialty Clinics
Hillcrest Medical Plaza
Appts: (309) 655-3889
Center Director: Umesh C. Chatrath, M.D.

Springfield—see Washington University CF Center (St. Louis, Missouri)

Urbana—see Washington University CF Center (St. Louis, Missouri)

INDIANA
Indianapolis
Cystic Fibrosis and Chronic Pulmonary Disease Center
Riley Hospital for Children
Indiana University Medical Center
Appts: (317) 274-7208
Center Director: Howard Eigen, M.D.
Adult Program Director: Veena Anthony, M.D.

Satellite Centers: Deaconess Hospital
Appts: (812) 426-3217
Parkview Memorial Hospital
Appts: (219) 484-6636 Ext. 41440
Director: Pushpom James, M.D.

South Bend
Cystic Fibrosis and Chronic Pulmonary Disease Clinic
St. Joseph's Medical Center
Appts: (800) 206-0879
Center Director: Edward A. Gergesha, M.D.
Associate Director: James Harris, M.D.

IOWA
Des Moines
Cystic Fibrosis Center
Blank Children's Hospital
Appts: (515) 241-8222
Center Director: Veljko Zivkovich, M.D.

Iowa City
Cystic Fibrosis Center
Pediatric Allergy and Pulmonary Division
Department of Pediatrics
University of Iowa Hospitals and Clinics
Appts: (319) 356-1853
Center Co-directors: Miles Weinberger, M.D., Richard Ahrens, M.D.

Satellite Center: McFarland Clinic
Mary Greeley Hospital
Appts: (515) 239-4482
Director: Edward G. Nassif, M.D.

KANSAS
Kansas City
Cystic Fibrosis Center
Kansas University Medical Center
Appts: (913) 588-6377
Center Director: Joseph Kanarek, M.D.
Center Co-director: Pam Shaw, M.D.

Wichita
Cystic Fibrosis Care and Teaching Center
Via Christi, St. Joseph Campus
Appts: (316) 689-4707
Center Director: Leonard L. Sullivan, M.D

KENTUCKY
Lexington
Cystic Fibrosis Center
Department of Pediatrics
Kentucky Clinic
Appts: (606) 323-8023
Center Director: Jamshed F.
Kanga, M.D.

Louisville
Kosair Children's Cystic Fibrosis
Center
Appts: (502) 629-8830
Center Director: Nemr Eid, M.D.

LOUISIANA
New Orleans
Tulane Cystic Fibrosis Center
Department of Pediatrics SL-37
Tulane University School of Medicine
Appts: (504) 587-7625
Center Director: Scott Davis, M.D.
Adult Program Director: Dean
Ellithorpe, M.D.

Shreveport
Cystic Fibrosis and Pediatric
Pulmonary Center
Louisiana State University Medical
Center
Appts: (318) 675-6094
Center Director: Bettina C. Hilman,
M.D.

MAINE
Bangor
Cystic Fibrosis Clinical Center
Eastern Maine Medical Center
Appts: (207) 973-7559
Center Director: Thomas Lever, M.D.

Lewiston
Central Maine Cystic Fibrosis Center
Central Maine Medical Center
Appts: (207) 795-2830
Center Director: Ralph V. Harder,
M.D.
Center Coordinator: Vernice Pelletier,
R.N.

Portland
Cystic Fibrosis Center
Maine Medical Center
Appts: (207) 871-2763
Center Director: Anne Marie Cairns,
D.O.
Associate Director: Nicholas K.
Fowler, M.D.
Associate Director: Jack Mann, M.D.
Adult Program Director: Edgar J.
Caldwell, M.D.

MARYLAND
Baltimore
The Johns Hopkins Hospital
Appts: (410) 955-2795
Center Director: Beryl J. Rosenstein,
M.D.
Adult Program Director: Sandra M.
Walden, M.D.

Bethesda
Cystic Fibrosis Center
National Institute of Diabetes and
Digestive and Kidney Diseases
National Institutes of Health
Appts: (301) 496-3434
Center Director: Milica S. Chernick,
M.D.

MASSACHUSETTS
Boston
Cystic Fibrosis Center
Pulmonary Division
Children's Hospital
Appts: (617) 355-7881
Center Director: Mary Ellen Wohl,
M.D.
Adult Program Director: Craig
Gerard, M.D.

Cystic Fibrosis Center
Massachusetts General Hospital
Appts: (617) 726-8707 or (617) 726-8708
Center Director: Allen Lapey, M.D.
Adult Program Director: Patricia M.
Joseph, M.D.

Cystic Fibrosis Center
Tufts New England Medical Center
Appts: (617) 636-5085
Center Director: Henry L. Dorkin,
M.D.

Springfield
Baystate Medical Center
Appts: (413) 784-2515
Center Director: Robert S. Gerstle,
M.D.

Worcester
University of Massachusetts Medical
Center
Department of Pediatrics
Appts: (508) 856-4155
Center Director: Robert G. Zwerdling,
M.D.

MICHIGAN
Ann Arbor
University of Michigan Cystic Fibrosis
Center
Appts: (313) 764-4123 (pediatrics),
(313) 936-5580 (adult)
Center Director: Samya Nasr, M.D.
Adult Program Director: Richard H.
Simon, M.D.

Detroit
Children's Hospital of Michigan
Cystic Fibrosis Care, Teaching and
Resource Center
Appts: (313) 745-5541
Center Director: Debbie Toder, M.D.

Adult Satellite Network: Wayne State
University
Harper Hospital
Appts: (313) 745-1735
Director: Dana Kissner, M.D.
Sinai Hospital of Detroit
Department of Medicine
Appts: (313) 493-6580
Director: Bohdan M. Pichurko, M.D.

Satellite Center: Mott Children's
Health Center
Appts: (810) 767-5750 Ext. 305
Director: H. Stephen Williams, M.D.,
M.P.H.

Grand Rapids
Butterworth Cystic Fibrosis Center
Appts: (616) 391-8890
Center Director: John Schuen, M.D.
Contact Person: Barbara Schoenborn,
R.N.

Kalamazoo
Michigan State University
Kalamazoo Center for Medical
Studies
Appts: (616) 337-6430
Center Director: Douglas N.
Homnick, M.D.

East Lansing
Michigan State University Cystic
Fibrosis Center
Appts: (517) 353-3241
Center Director: Richard E. Honicky,
M.D.

MINNESOTA
Minneapolis
University of Minnesota
Appts: (612) 624-0962
Center Director: Warren J. Warwick,
M.D.

MISSISSIPPI
Jackson
University of Mississippi Medical
Center
Department of Pediatrics
Appts: (601) 984-5205
Center Director: Suzanne T. Miller,
M.D.

MISSOURI
Columbia
Columbia Cystic Fibrosis, Pediatric
Pulmonary and Gastrointestinal
Center
University of Missouri Medical Center
Department of Child Health
Appts: (573) 882-6921
Center Director: Peter König, M.D.

Outreach Clinics: St. John's Regional
Hospital
Appts: (573) 882-6978
Contact: Kelly Moore, R.N., M.S.
Southeast Missouri Hospital
Appts: (573) 651-5550
Contact: Kelly Moore, R.N., M.S.

Kansas City
The Children's Mercy Hospital
University of Missouri, Kansas City
School of Medicine
Pediatric Pulmonology Section
Appts: (816) 234-3066
Sweat Test Only: (816) 234-3230
Center Director: Michael McCubbin,
M.D.

St. Louis
Cystic Fibrosis, Pediatric Pulmonary
and Pediatric Gastrointestinal
Center
Cardinal Glennon Memorial Hospital
for Children
Appts: (314) 577-5663
Center Director: Anthony J. Rejent,
M.D.
Adult Program Director: Mary Ellen
Kleinhenz, M.D., St. Louis
University Medical Center

Washington University School of
Medicine Cystic Fibrosis Center
Appts: (314) 454-2694, (314) 362-9366
(adults), (314) 454-6248 (sweat test
only)
Center Director: George B.
Mallory, Jr., M.D.
Pediatric Coordinator: Jane A.
Quaute, R.N., B.S.
Adult Program Director: Daniel
Rosenbluth, M.D.
Adult Coordinator: Sharon Muhs,
B.S.N.

Satellite Centers: Southern Illinois
University School of Medicine
Appts: (217) 782-0187 Ext. 2321 or
(217) 788-3381
Director: Lanie E. Eagleton, M.D.
Coordinator: Joni Colle, R.N., R.R.T.
Carle Clinic Association
Appts: (217) 383-3100
Director: Donald F. Davison, M.D.

MONTANA: See Denver, Colorado

NEBRASKA
Omaha
Nebraska Regional Center for Cystic
Fibrosis and Pediatric Pulmonary
Diseases
University of Nebraska Medical
Center
Appts: (402) 559-4156
Center Director: John L. Colombo,
M.D.

NEVADA
Las Vegas
Children's Lung Specialists
Appts: (702) 598-4411
Center Director: Ruben Diaz, M.D.

NEW HAMPSHIRE
Hanover/Manchester
New Hampshire Cystic Fibrosis Care,
Research and Teaching Center
Dartmouth Hitchcock Medical
Center
Appts: (603) 650-6244 (Lebanon) or
(603) 695-2560 (Bedford)
Center Director: William Boyle, Jr.,
M.D.

NEW JERSEY
Newark
New Jersey Medical School
Appts: (201) 982-4815
Center Director: Nelson L. Turcios,
M.D.

Satellite Center: Cystic Fibrosis
Center
Hackensack Medical Center
Appts: (201) 996-2121
Director: Lawrence J. Denson, M.D.

Long Branch
Cystic Fibrosis and Pediatric
Pulmonary Center
Monmouth Medical Center
Appts: (908) 222-4474
Center Director: Robert L. Zanni,
M.D.

NEW MEXICO
Albuquerque
University of New Mexico School of
Medicine
Department of Pediatrics
Appts: (505) 272-6633
Center Acting Director: Bennie C.
McWilliams, M.D.

NEW YORK
Albany
Pediatric Pulmonary and Cystic
Fibrosis Center
Albany Medical College
Appts: (518) 262-6880
Center Director: Robert A. Kaslovsky,
M.D.
Adult Program Director: Jonathan M.
Rosen, M.D.

Brooklyn
Long Island College Hospital
Appts: (718) 780-1025 or
(718) 780-1026
Center Director: Robert Giusti, M.D.
Outreach Clinic: St. Vincent's Medical
Center of Richmond

Buffalo
Children's Lung and Cystic Fibrosis
Center
Children's Hospital of Buffalo
Appts: (716) 878-7524
Center Director: Drucy Borowitz,
M.D.
Adult Program Director: Colin
McMahon, M.D.

New Hyde Park
Cystic Fibrosis and Pediatric
Pulmonary Center
Schneider Children's Hospital of
Long Island
Jewish Medical Center
Albert Einstein College of Medicine
Appts: (718) 470-3250
Center Director: Jack D. Gorvoy,
M.D.

Satellite Center: Good Samaritan
Hospital Medical Center
Appts: (516) 376-4191
Director: Louis E. Guida, Jr., M.D.
Associate Director: Joseph S.
Chiamonte, M.D.

New York City
Cystic Fibrosis and Pediatric
    Pulmonary Center
Mount Sinai School of Medicine
Appts: (212) 241-7788
Center Director: Richard J. Bonforte,
    M.D.

Pediatric Pulmonary Center, BHS 101
Babies Hospital and Columbia
    Presbyterian Medical Center
Appts: (212) 305-5122
Center Director: Lynne M. Quittell,
    M.D.

Cystic Fibrosis, Pediatric Pulmonary
    and Gastrointestinal Center
St. Vincent's Hospital and Medical
    Center of New York
Appts: (212) 604-8895 or (212) 604-8898
Center Director: Joan DeCelie-
    Germana, M.D.

Rochester
University of Rochester Medical
    Center
Strong Memorial Hospital
Department of Pediatrics
Appts: (716) 275-2464
Center Director: Karen Z. Voter,
    M.D.

Satellite Center: House of the Good
    Samaritan
Appts: (315) 788-2211
Director: Ronald Perciaccante, M.D.

Stony Brook
University Medical Center at Stony
    Brook
Department of Pediatrics
Appts: (516) 444-7726
Center Director: Clement Ren, M.D.

Syracuse
Robert C. Schwartz Cystic Fibrosis
    Center
University Hospital
SUNY Health Science Center
Appts: (315) 473-5834
Center Directors: Ran Anbar,
    M.D.and Debra Iannuzzi, M.D.

Valhalla
The Armond V. Mascia Cystic Fibrosis
    Center
New York Medical College
Appts: (914) 285-7585
Center Director: Allen Dozor, M.D.

NORTH CAROLINA
Chapel Hill
U.N.C. Cystic Fibrosis Center
University of North Carolina
Department of Pediatrics, CB #7220
Appts: (919) 966-1055 (pediatrics),
    (919) 966-1077 (adults-18 years and
    older)
Center Director: Gerald W. Fernald,
    M.D.

Adult Program: Cystic Fibro-
    sis/Pulmonary Research and
    Training Center
The University of North Carolina at
    Chapel Hill
Director: Michael Knowles, M.D.

Satellite Center: The Children's
    Hospital at Carolinas Medical
    Center
Children's Respiratory Center
Appts: (704) 355-1130
Director: Bill Ashe, M.D.

Durham
Cystic Fibrosis and Pediatric
    Pulmonary Center
Duke University Medical Center
Appts: (919) 684-3364
Center Director: Marc Majure, M.D.
Center Co-director: Thomas Murphy,
    M.D.
Adult Center Co-director: Peter S.
    Kussin, M.D.

Satellite Center: Pediatric Pulmonary
    Medicine, P.A.
Director: Jane V. Gwinn, M.D.

NORTH DAKOTA
Bismarck
Cystic Fibrosis Center
St. Alexius Medical Center
Appts: (701) 224-7500
Center Director: Allan Stillerman,
    M.D.

OHIO
Akron
Lewis H. Walker, M.D. Cystic Fibrosis
    Center
Children's Hospital Medical Center
    of Akron
Appts: (330) 379-8545
Center Director: Robert T. Stone,
    M.D.

Cincinnati
The Children's Hospital Medical
    Center
Pulmonary Medicine
Department of Pediatrics
Appts: (513) 559-6771 (ask for Jeanne
    Weiland, R.N.)
Center Director: Robert Wilmott,
    M.D.
Adult Program Director: Janine
    Mylett, M.D., University of
    Cincinnati

Cleveland
The Leroy Matthews Cystic Fibrosis
    Center
Rainbow Babies and Childrens
    Hospital/University Hospitals of
    Cleveland
Case Western Reserve University
    School of Medicine
Appts: (216) 844-3267
Center Director: Carl F. Doershuk,
    M.D.

Columbus
Cystic Fibrosis Center
Columbus Children's Hospital
Appts: (614) 722-4766
Center Director: Karen S. McCoy,
    M.D.

Dayton
Pediatric Pulmonary Center
The Children's Medical Center
Appts: (513) 226-8376
Center Director: Michael E. Steffan,
    M.D.

OKLAHOMA
Children's Hospital of Oklahoma
University of Oklahoma
Health Science Center
Appts: (405) 271-6390
Center Director: John E. Grunow,
    M.D.

OREGON
Portland
Cystic Fibrosis Care, Teaching and
    Research Center
Appts: (503) 494-8023
Center Director: Michael Wall, M.D.
Outreach Clinic: Medford CF Clinic,
    Rogue Valley Hospital

PENNSYLVANIA
Harrisburg
Cystic Fibrosis Center
Pinnacle Health at Polyclinic Medical
Center
Appts: (717) 782-4105
Center Director: Muttiah
Ganeshananthan, M.D.

Philadelphia
Cystic Fibrosis Center for Care,
Teaching and Research
The Children's Hospital of
Philadelphia
University of Pennsylvania School of
Medicine
Appts: (215) 590-3749/3510 (Mon.
through Fri. 8:30–4:30; evenings
and weekends, ask for physician
on call)
Center Director: Thomas F. Scanlin,
M.D.

Adult Program: Department of
Medicine
Pulmonary Medicine/Critical Care
Medicine
Hospital of the University of
Pennsylvania
Appts: (215) 662-3202
Director: Cynthia Robinson, M.D.

The Medical College of
Pennsylvania/Hahnemann
University School of Medicine
St. Christopher's Hospital for
Children
Appts: (215) 427-5183
Center Director: Daniel V. Schidlow,
M.D.

Adult Program: Pulmonary Disease
and Critical Care
Medical College of Pennsylvania
Hospital
Appts: (215) 842-7748
Director: Stanley Fiel, M.D.
Outreach Clinic: Mercy Hospital

Pittsburgh
Cystic Fibrosis Center
Children's Hospital of Pittsburgh
University of Pittsburgh School of
Medicine
Appts: (412) 692-5630
Center Director: David M. Orenstein,
M.D.
Adult Program Director: Joel
Weinberg, M.D.

PUERTO RICO
San Juan
Cystic Fibrosis Care and Teaching
Center
Pediatric Pulmonary Program
Department of Pediatrics
University of Puerto Rico
Medical Sciences Campus
Appts: (809) 754-3733 or (809) 754-3722
Center Director: Jose Rodriguez
Santana, M.D.

RHODE ISLAND
Providence
Cystic Fibrosis Center
Rhode Island Hospital
Appts: (401) 444-5685
Center Director: Mary Ann Passero,
M.D.

SOUTH CAROLINA
Charleston
Cystic Fibrosis Center
Medical University of South Carolina
Appts: (803) 792-3561
Center Director: Robert D. Baker,
M.D., Ph.D.
Adult Program Director: Patrick
Flume, M.D.

SOUTH DAKOTA
Sioux Falls
South Dakota Cystic Fibrosis Center
Sioux Valley Hospital
Appts: (605) 333-7189
Center Director: Rodney R. Parry,
M.D.

TENNESSEE
Memphis
Memphis Cystic Fibrosis Center
Le Bonheur Children's Medical
   Center
University of Tennessee Center for
   the Health Sciences
Appts: (901) 572-5222
Center Director: Robert
   Schoumacher, M.D.

Nashville
Cystic Fibrosis Care Teaching and
   Research Center
Vanderbilt University Medical Center
Appts: (615) 343-7617
Center Director: Preston W.
   Campbell, M.D.
Adult Program Director: Angelo
   Canonico, M.D.
Phone: (615) 343-7617

Satellite Centers: East Tennessee
   Children's Hospital
Appts: (615) 541-8336
Director: Don Ellenburg, M.D.
Co-director: John Rogers, M.D.
T.C. Thompson Children's Hospital
Appts: (615) 778-6505
Director: Joel Ledbetter, M.D.

TEXAS
Dallas
Cystic Fibrosis Care, Teaching and
   Research Center
Children's Medical Center
Appts: (214) 640-2361 or (214) 640-2362
Center Director: Claude Prestidge,
   M.D.

Adult Program: St. Paul Medical
   Center
Director: Randall Rosenblatt, M.D.

Satellite Centers: Permian Basin
   Allergy Center
Allergy Alliances
Appts: (915) 561-8183
Director: John D. Bray, M.D.
Scott & White Clinic
Appts: (817) 724-4950
Director: James F. Daniel, M.D.
Tulsa Ambulatory Pediatric Center
Appts: (918) 838-4820
Director: John C. Kramer, M.D.
The University of Texas Health
   Center at Tyler
Appts: (903) 877-7220
Director: Robert B. Klein, M.D.

Fort Sam Houston
Tri-Services Military CF Center
Pulmonary/Critical Care Medicine
   Department
Wilford Hal USAF Medical Center
Appts: (210) 670-7347
Center Co-directors: Dr. Stephen
   Inscore, LTC, MC, USA, Dr. Jan
Westerman, MAJ., MC, USAF

Satellite Centers: Naval Hospital San
   Diego
Department of Pediatrics
Appts: (619) 532-6896
Director: B. Gaston, CDR
Tripler Army Medical Center
Department of Pediatrics
Appts: (808) 433-6407
Director: Dr. Charles Callahan, MAJ,
   MC
National Naval Medical Center
Appts: (301) 295-4902 or (301) 295-4903
Director: Dr. Donna Perry, CAPT,
   MC, USN
Clinic Coordinator: Jane A. Dean,
   R.N.

USAF Medical Center Keesler
Appts: (601) 377-6620
Director: Dr. James Woodward, MAJ,
    USAF
William Beaumont Army Medical
    Center
Department of Pediatrics
Appts: (915) 569-2000
Director: Dr. Larry Tremper, LTC,
    MC, USA
Portsmouth Naval Medical Center
Appts: (804) 398-7558 (DSN 564)
Director: John Pfaff, CDR, MC,
    USNR
Madigan Army Medical Center
Department of Pediatrics
Appts: (206) 968-1980 or (206) 968-3333
Director: Dr. Donald Moffitt, COL,
    MC, USA

Fort Worth
Cystic Fibrosis Center
Cook-Ft. Worth Children's Medical
    Center
Appts: (817) 885-4202
Center Co-director: James C.
    Cunningham, M.D.
Center Co-director: Nancy Dambro,
    M.D.

Outreach Clinic: Texas Tech
    University Health Sciences Center
Appts: (806) 354-5613
Co-directors: James C. Cunningham,
    M.D., Maynard Dyson, M.D.

Houston
Cystic Fibrosis Center
Pulmonology Section
Department of Pediatrics
Baylor College of Medicine
Appts: (713) 770-3013
Center Director: Peter W. Hiatt, M.D.
Adult Program Director: Kathryn
    Hale, M.D.
Phone: (714) 790-2076

Satellite Center: Seton Medical Center
Appts: (512) 454-3387
Director: Allan L. Frank, M.D.

San Antonio
Cystic Fibrosis-Chronic Lung Disease
    Center
Santa Rosa Children's Hospital
Appts: (210) 228-2058 or (210) 228-2201
Center Co-directors: Amanda Dove,
    M.D., Humberto A. Hidalgo,
    M.D.

UTAH
Salt Lake City
Intermountain Cystic Fibrosis Center
Department of Pediatrics
University of Utah Medical Center
Appts: (801) 588-2621 (pediatrics),
    (801) 581-2410 (adults)
Center Co-directors: Dennis Nielson,
    M.D., Ph.D., Bruce C. Marshall,
    M.D. (adult program)

Satellite Centers: Mercy Medical
    Center
Appts: (208) 463-3190
Director: Eugene M. Brown, M.D.
Pocatello, ID
Appts: (208) 232-1443
Director: Don McInturff, M.D.
Idaho Falls, ID
Appts: (208) 523-3060
Director: George H. Groberg, M.D.

VERMONT
Burlington
Cystic Fibrosis and Pediatric
    Pulmonary Center
Appts: (802) 862-5529
Center Director: Donald R. Swartz,
    M.D.

VIRGINIA
Charlottesville
Cystic Fibrosis Care, Teaching and Research Center
University of Virginia School of Medicine
Appts: (804) 924-2250
Center Director: Robert F. Selden, Jr., M.D.
Adult Program Director: Mark Robbins, M.D.
Phone: (804) 924-9687

Norfolk
Eastern Virginia Medical School
Children's Hospital of the King's Daughters
Appts: (804) 668-7132
Center Director: Thomas Rubio, M.D.
Associate Director: Karl Karlson, M.D.
Adult Program Director: Ignacio Ripoll, M.D.

Richmond
Cystic Fibrosis Program
Medical College of Virginia
Appts: (804) 786-9445
Center Director: David A. Draper, M.D.

WASHINGTON
Seattle
Pulmonary Disease and Cystic Fibrosis Center
Children's Hospital and Medical Center
Appts: (206) 526-2024
Center Director: Bonnie W. Ramsey, M.D.

Adult Program: Cystic Fibrosis Clinic
Division of Pulmonary and Critical Care Medicine
University of Washington Medical Center
Appts: (206) 548-4615
Clinic Coordinator: Gwen McDonald, R.N., M.S.
Director: Moira Aitken, M.D.

Satellite Centers: Anchorage Cystic Fibrosis Clinic
Providence Hospital
Appts: (907) 561-5440
Director: Dion Roberts, M.D.
Mary Bridge Children's Health Center
Appts: (206) 552-1415
Co-directors: Lawrence A. Larson, D.O., David Ricker, M.D.
Deaconess Medical Center
Appts: (509) 458-7300
Director: Michael M. McCarthy, M.D.

WEST VIRGINIA
Morgantown
Mountain State Cystic Fibrosis Center
Robert C. Byrd Health Science Center
West Virginia University School of Medicine
Appts: (304) 293-1841
Center Director: Stephen C. Aronoff, M.D.

WISCONSIN
Madison
University of Wisconsin
Cystic Fibrosis/Pediatric Pulmonary Center
Appts: (608) 263-8555
Center Director: Michael J. Rock, M.D.

Adult Program: University of
  Wisconsin
Adult Cystic Fibrosis Program
Appts: (608) 263-7203
Adult Program Director: Guillermo A.
  doPico, M.D.
Adult Nurse Coordinator: Lorna Will,
  R.N., M.A.

Milwaukee
Children's Hospital of Wisconsin, MS
  #777A
Medical College of Wisconsin
Cystic Fibrosis Clinic
Appts: (414) 266-6730
Center Director: Mark Splaingard,
  M.D.
Adult Program Director: Julie A.
  Biller, M.D.

For more information or to find more contact information
about a treatment center in your area, call the Cystic Fibrosis
Foundation in Maryland at 1-800-FIGHT-CF.

Glossary

ABC proteins A large family of proteins containing an ATP-binding cassette; the CFTR channel is a member of this protein family.

Acinar cells Cells in the pancreas that produce digestive enzymes and secrete them into small ducts that eventually empty into the small intestine.

Adenovirus A virus that causes the common cold; scientists use a modified version of this virus to introduce the CFTR gene into airway cells in CF patients who are participating in gene-therapy trials.

Aerosol A fine mist that contains liquid or solid particles of a medicine that can be inhaled; doctors sometimes use this method to administer antibiotics to people with CF.

Allele One of the possible forms of a particular gene.

Alveoli Tiny, thin-walled sacs that bud from the ends of the bronchioles in the lung; alveoli associate with capillaries and serve as the site for the exchange of oxygen and carbon dioxide between inhaled air and the blood.

Amino acids The building blocks from which proteins are made.

Aminoglycosides A type of antibiotic that kills or inhibits the growth of bacteria by interfering with their ability to synthesize proteins.

Amniocentesis Removal of a small quantity of amniotic fluid and cells from within the uterus during pregnancy, usually for the purpose of performing genetic tests on the fetus.

Amylase An enzyme found in saliva which breaks down starch into polysaccharides and disaccharides.

Antibiotics Any chemical that can kill or inhibit the growth or activity of a microbe; antibiotics are selectively toxic, affecting bacteria but not the infected host.

Aspergillus A common fungus that sometimes infects people with CF.

Asthma A reversible constriction of the airways, characterized by wheezing and difficulty in breathing; asthma can be caused by allergies and is a disorder separate from CF.

ATP Adenosine triphosphate, an energy-rich molecule that provides fuel for many cellular activities.

Beta defensin A natural antibiotic that may be produced by the epithelial cells lining the lungs; the molecule appears to be disabled by the high salt concentrations present in the lungs of people with CF.

Bile A fluid produced by the liver, stored in the gall bladder, and secreted into the intestines; helps digest fats.

Bronchi The two major branches of the trachea that lead to the lungs.

Bronchiectasis Chronic weakening and widening of the bronchial walls, often due to infection and poor drainage of mucus.

Bronchiolitis Inflammation of the finer branches of the bronchial tree; associated with respiratory distress and wheezing.

Bronchitis Acute or chronic inflammation of the lining of the trachea and bronchi.

Bronchodilator Drug capable of dilating bronchial tubes and relieving bronchospasm.

Bronchospasm A temporary spasm or contraction of the bronchi.

Button gastrostomy A surgical procedure that involves inserting a small tube into the stomach; allows patients who cannot gain weight to receive night feedings of high-calorie mixtures of proteins and fats.

Carbohydrates Organic compounds made of carbon, hydrogen, and oxygen that provide a major source of energy for the body; carbohydrates include simple sugars, such as glucose, and more complex sugars, such as sucrose (common table sugar).

Carbon dioxide A gas produced by animals' cells during respiration.

Carrier A person who possesses one copy of a gene that in a double dose could cause a disease; such a "heterozygous" individual carries a defective allele but does not suffer from the disease.

Cervix The narrow opening that links the vagina with the uterus; the cervix is covered by mucus-producing epithelial cells.

CFTR The cystic fibrosis transmembrane conductance regulator—the protein made by the gene responsible for CF; the CFTR protein is thought to act as an ion channel that permits chloride to enter and exit certain epithelial cells.

Cholera An infectious disease that causes severe diarrhea, electrolyte imbalances, and rapid loss of body fluid; scientists think that a mutant CFTR gene might protect carriers from cholera.

Chloride ion The negatively charged portion of a molecule of many salts, including sodium chloride (common table salt).

Chorionic villus The outer surface of the membrane that surrounds a developing fetus; a piece of this membrane can be removed for prenatal diagnosis of CF and other diseases.

Chromosomes The threadlike structures in the cell that carry the genes.

Chymotrypsin Digestive enzyme secreted by the pancreas; breaks proteins into peptides and amino acids.

Cilia Tiny, hairlike structures present on the surface of epithelial cells, including those that line the airways of the lungs.

Cirrhosis Chronic scarring and destruction of the liver.

Clubbing An enlargement of the tips of the fingers and toes; the cause is unknown, but clubbing is associated with chronic lung disease.

Codon Three nucleotide bases, which, when read by the cellular machinery, encode a single amino acid in a protein.

Congenital bilateral absence of the vas deferens (CBAVD) Complete absence of the vas deferens at birth.

Creon An enzyme supplement taken by people with CF; contains lipase, amylase, and protease to help in digestion of fats, sugars, and proteins.

Cystic fibrosis of the pancreas The original name of CF; characterized by scarring of the cysts present in the pancreas.

ΔF508 The most common CFTR mutation found in the white population; the mutation dictates the formation of a CFTR protein missing one amino acid—the phenylalanine (F) at position 508.

Diabetes A chronic disease characterized by increased levels of sugar in the blood; destruction of the insulin-producing cells in the pancreas sometimes causes diabetes in people with CF.

DNA Deoxyribonucleic acid—the biological molecule that carries the genetic information in a cell; genes are made of DNA.

DNase A drug that digests DNA; can be inhaled by patients with CF to help keep the airways clear of the long, sticky strands of DNA that can thicken mucus.

Dominant A genetic trait that is expressed in a heterozygote.

Ducts Tubular passages through which secretions are carried.

Electrolytes A solution of salts.

Emphysema Enlargement of the air sacs in the lungs; causes labored breathing and increased susceptibility to infection.

Endocrine glands Ductless glands such as the pituitary and adrenal glands, which secrete their products directly into the bloodstream.

Endoplasmic reticulum A complex network of membranes in the cell cytoplasm that participates in protein synthesis and processing.

Enzyme A protein, produced by living cells, capable of performing specific chemical reactions.

Epithelial cells Cells that form a layer covering or lining surfaces within the body, including organs such as the lung, pancreas, and sweat glands.

Exocrine glands Glands such as the pancreas, sweat glands, and gall bladder, which secrete their products into ducts.

Exon The part of a gene that codes for an RNA or protein product.

Fats Organic compounds composed of carbon, hydrogen, and oxygen; important fuel for the body and part of cell membranes.

Fibrosis Replacement of important parts of a tissue with scarring.

Flimm fighter A mechanical percussor used by people with CF during physiotherapy to help dislodge mucus from the lungs.

Flutter A physiotherapy aide that helps loosen mucus in the lungs of people with CF.

Gamete A mature reproductive cell—sperm or egg.

Gene therapy Experimental procedure that provides cells with a functional copy of a gene that may be missing or defective.

Genes The fundamental unit of heredity; the coding region of DNA.

Genome All the genetic information of an individual.

Heat stroke Sudden and severe attack of headache, dizziness, and cramps often caused by excessive loss of salt through the sweat in hot weather or during a high fever.

Heterozygote An individual who has two different forms of a gene; see also **carrier**.

Homozygote An individual who has identical alleles for a particular gene.

Huffing Quick, forced exhalations that help to clear the lungs of mucus during physiotherapy.

Ileum The lower portion of the small intestine.

Immunreactive trypsinogen A molecular marker that is elevated in the blood of newborns with CF.

Immunosuppressant Drugs that suppress the body's immune response against foreign tissues or proteins; given after transplants to prevent rejection of the new organ.

In vitro fertilization Fertilization of an egg by a sperm in the laboratory.

Introns Bits of DNA sequence that separate the coding exons in genes.

Ion A charged particle.

Ion channel A molecular gate in the cell membrane through which ions pass into or out of the cell.

Jaundice Yellowish discoloration of skin or tissues caused by a blockage that stops bile from traveling from the liver to the intestine.

Linkage analysis A method for finding the location of a gene on a chromosome by analyzing the inheritance of markers that lie nearby.

Lipase An enzyme that digests fats.

Lipids Fats.

Liposome A small vesicle made of fat particles; used to deliver genes to cells in some experimental gene therapy protocols.

Malabsorption Impaired absorption of nutrients from the small intestine into the body.

Malnutrition Any disorder that results from inappropriate dietary intake or improper processing of nutrients.

Meconium ileus Obstruction of the small intestine by fetal excrement at birth.

Meconium ileus equivalent Intestinal obstruction in older patients; also called distal intestinal obstruction syndrome.

Messenger RNA A molecule that carries genetic information from the DNA in the nucleus to the cytoplasm, where the cellular machinery translates its information into the amino-acid sequence of a protein.

Microvilli Tiny, fingerlike projections that line the small intestine and increase the surface area available for the absorption of nutrients into the blood.

Mucus A suspension of glycoproteins, water, cells, and salts secreted as a lubricant that coats and protects the lining of some glands; thickened in patients with CF.

Mutation A permanent and heritable mistake in a gene.

Nasal polyps Benign growths in the nasal linings; caused by enlargement and blockage of mucous glands.

Nebulizer An apparatus that converts a liquid into a fine mist for inhalation.

Neutrophils Immune cells that can kill and engulf microbes.

Nucleic acids DNA and RNA.

Nucleotides The building blocks of DNA and RNA.

Nutrizym An enzyme supplement taken by people with CF; contains lipase, amylase, and protease to help in digestion of fats, sugars, and proteins.

Oxygen A gas of which one-fifth of the earth's atmosphere is composed; most organisms require oxygen to efficiently produce ATP, the molecule that supplies the cell with a source of energy.

Pan-resistant *Pseudomonas* A strain of bacteria that is resistant to most of the commonly used antibiotics; infection with pan-resistant bacteria may disqualify a patient with CF for a lung transplant.

Pancrease An enzyme supplement taken by people with CF; contains lipase, amylase, and protease to help in digestion of fats, sugars, and proteins.

Pancreatic insufficiency Loss of pancreas function in 85 percent of patients with CF, caused by the accumulation of thickened mucus which blocks the ducts that carry digestive enzymes from the pancreas to the small intestine.

Penicillin Widely used antibiotic that kills bacteria by inhibiting their synthesis of a cell wall.

Percussion Vigorous clapping or thumping on the chest or back of a person with CF; helps to dislodge mucus from the lungs during physiotherapy.

Phosphatase An enzyme that removes phosphate groups from proteins.

Phosphorylation A chemical modification—addition of a phosphate group—that regulates the activity of a protein.

Physiotherapy Thumping on the chest and back of a person with CF to dislodge and drain mucus from lungs; usually performed two or three times each day.

Pneumothorax Air trapped in the chest cavity outside the lungs; prevents the normal movement of lungs during breathing.

Postural drainage The assisted movement of mucus from the lungs through a combination of chest percussion and appropriate positioning of the person with CF; also called bronchial drainage.

Pseudomonas aeruginosa Species of bacterium most frequently isolated from the sputum of people with CF; *Pseudomonas* can be more difficult to eradicate than other respiratory infections.

Pulmozyme DNase produced by Genentech, Inc.

Recessive Trait expressed only in the homozygote; CF is a recessive disease.

Rectal prolapse Protrusion of the rectum through the anus.

Respiratory failure Impairment of the exchange of oxygen and carbon dioxide between inhaled air and the blood.

RNA Ribonucleic acid; functions as the middleman in the translation of DNA to protein.

Sinusitis Inflammation of the linings of the air-filled cavities inside the head.

Spirometer Instrument for measuring the amount of air breathed into and out of the lungs.

Sputum Phlegm coughed up from the airway passages.

Staphylococcus aureus A common bacterium associated with lung infections in people with CF.

Sweat test Determination of the concentration of chloride in sweat; the most reliable diagnostic test for CF.

Trachea The large tube that carries air into the bronchi.

Trypsin An enzyme, secreted by the pancreas, which digests proteins.

UTP Uridine triphosphate—a drug that may stimulate the activity of alternative chloride-ion channels in the lungs of people with CF.

Vas deferens Tube that connects the testes with the prostate gland, where sperm mixes with the other components of semen; the vas deferens is usually missing in males with CF.

Xenotransplantation Transplantation of animal organs into a human.

Index

PLEASE SHARE YOUR THOUGHTS ON THIS BOOK

comments:	comments:
comments:	comments:
comments:	comments:
comments:	comments:
comments:	comments:
comments:	comments: